AF515883

# PERITONEAL DIALYSIS CAREGIVER GUIDE

*Complete Home Care Manual for Patients, Attendants & Family Caregivers*

*Gerard Assey*

**PERITONEAL DIALYSIS CAREGIVER GUIDE:**

*Complete Home Care Manual for Patients, Attendants & Family Caregivers*

By

**Gerard Assey**

© Copyright 2026 by Author

*Published by:*
Gerard Assey
19/18, Palli Arasan Street
Anna Nagar East
Chennai - 600 102

**ISBN:** 978-81-998781-8-1

All Rights Reserved. No part of this publication may be reproduced, stored in a retrieval system, or transmitted in any form or by any means- electronic or mechanical, including photocopying, recording, or by any information storage and retrieval system, without prior written permission from the author.

# DISCLAIMER

The information provided in this book, "**PERITONEAL DIALYSIS CAREGIVER GUIDE: *Complete Home Care Manual for Patients, Attendants & Family Caregivers***," is based on personal caregiving experience, practical learning, and publicly available knowledge related to peritoneal dialysis home care.
The author is not a medical doctor, nephrologist, dialysis nurse, or licensed healthcare professional. This book is not intended to replace professional medical advice, diagnosis, or treatment.
All medical decisions, treatment changes, medication adjustments, dialysis prescriptions, and emergency responses must be made strictly under the guidance of a qualified healthcare provider.

Readers are strongly advised to:

- ✓ *Consult their nephrologist or dialysis team before implementing any procedure described in this book.*
- ✓ *Follow the official training provided by their dialysis center.*
- ✓ *Refer to manufacturer instructions for medical equipment.*
- ✓ *Seek immediate medical attention in case of complications or emergencies.*

While every effort has been made to present accurate and practical information, medical knowledge and protocols may change over time. The author and publisher assume no responsibility or liability for any injury, loss, damage, or adverse outcome resulting from the use or misuse of the information contained in this book.

This guide is intended solely as a supportive educational resource for caregivers and families, and not as a substitute for professional medical training or clinical supervision.

By reading and using this book, the reader acknowledges full responsibility for their own medical decisions and agrees to consult qualified healthcare professionals for individualized care.

# PREFACE

Peritoneal Dialysis (PD) is more than a medical procedure — it is a daily rhythm of life that enters the home, reshapes routines, and transforms family members into caregivers.

This book was not written from a hospital desk, but from lived experience.

When kidney failure entered our home, it brought fear, uncertainty, technical terms, sterile procedures, and endless questions. Yet alongside the challenges came knowledge, discipline, courage, and a deep understanding that informed caregiving can restore confidence and stability in even the most fragile moments.

As a husband and primary caregiver walking closely through my wife's PD journey, I discovered that families often receive instructions — but not always clarity. They are shown procedures — but not always the reasoning behind them. They are trained technically — but not prepared emotionally.

This guide is written to bridge that gap.

It is designed to simplify complex medical processes into practical, step-by-step understanding for patients, attendants, and family caregivers. It aims to build competence, reduce anxiety, prevent avoidable mistakes, and help caregivers feel equipped rather than overwhelmed.

Peritoneal Dialysis, when managed correctly, allows patients to live with dignity, flexibility, and hope. Home-based care becomes safe and sustainable when caregivers understand not just *what* to do, but *why* they are doing it.

This manual does not replace professional medical advice. Rather, it complements it — reinforcing best practices, encouraging vigilance, and promoting responsible care.

If this book helps even one family feel more confident, more prepared, and more at peace in their PD journey, it has fulfilled its purpose.

May it serve as a steady companion in your caregiving path.

# ACKNOWLEDGEMENT

This book has been shaped not only by experience gained, but also from the learning, guidance and support of the dedicated medical professionals who walked alongside us during a challenging season of life.

I wish to express my sincere gratitude to Dr. R. Balasubramaniyam, Chief Nephrologist; Dr. Balaji Kirushnan, Senior Consultant, other Doctors, Ms. Sasikala, Nephro Manager, and the entire Peritoneal Dialysis and Hemodialysis team at Kauvery Hospital.

Their professionalism, patience, clinical excellence, and genuine concern for my wife's well-being made an immense difference in our journey. Beyond medical care, they offered reassurance, clarity, and compassion during moments of uncertainty.

This acknowledgement is offered purely as a personal expression of appreciation. The content of this book reflects my individual experience as a caregiver and does not represent the official views or endorsement of the above-mentioned doctors, team, or institution.

With gratitude and respect.

# Table of Contents

# PART 1:
# UNDERSTANDING PERITONEAL DIALYSIS

# Chapter 1: Understanding Kidney Failure & Why PD is Needed

When someone in the family is told that their kidneys are not working properly, life changes overnight. There are new words, new routines, new fears — and many questions.

This chapter will help you understand, in simple language, what is happening inside the body and why Peritoneal Dialysis (PD) becomes necessary. The more you understand, the more confident and calm you will feel as a caregiver.

**What Do the Kidneys Do?**

Most people do not think about their kidneys — until something goes wrong.

We all have two kidneys, located at the back of the abdomen, one on each side of the spine. Each kidney is about the size of a fist. Though small, they perform powerful life-saving functions every single day.

The kidneys act like the body's natural filter.

Here is what they do:

1. Remove Waste from the Blood

Every time we eat, drink, or take medicines, the body produces waste. The kidneys filter the blood and remove these waste products through urine.

If waste is not removed, it builds up in the body and becomes poisonous.

2. Remove Extra Water

The kidneys balance how much water stays in the body. If you drink more fluids, they remove the extra.

If you drink less, they conserve water. Without this balance, swelling, breathlessness, or dehydration can occur.

3. Maintain Salt and Mineral Balance

The kidneys regulate sodium, potassium, calcium, and other minerals. If potassium rises too high, it can affect the heart rhythm — which can be life-threatening.

4. Control Blood Pressure

The kidneys help regulate blood pressure. Damaged kidneys often lead to high blood pressure — and high blood pressure further damages the kidneys. It becomes a dangerous cycle.

5. Help Make Red Blood Cells

The kidneys produce a hormone that tells the body to make red blood cells. When kidneys fail, patients often feel tired and weak due to anemia.

When kidneys stop doing these jobs properly, the body slowly fills with waste and extra fluid. That is when medical help becomes urgent.

**Acute vs Chronic Kidney Failure**

Not all kidney problems are the same. It is important to understand the difference.

**Acute Kidney Failure (Sudden Kidney Injury)**

This happens suddenly — sometimes within hours or days.

Common causes:

- ✓ *Severe infection*
- ✓ *Dehydration*
- ✓ *Major surgery*
- ✓ *Certain medicines*
- ✓ *Severe drop in blood pressure*

The good news: In many cases, acute kidney failure can improve if treated quickly. Dialysis may be temporary.

**Chronic Kidney Disease (CKD)**

This develops slowly over months or years.

Common causes:

- ✓ *Diabetes*
- ✓ *High blood pressure*
- ✓ *Long-standing kidney infections*
- ✓ *Genetic conditions*

In chronic kidney disease, the damage usually cannot be reversed. Over time, kidney function decreases permanently.

When kidney function falls below a critical level (usually around 10–15% function remaining), dialysis or transplant becomes necessary to survive.

This stage is called **End-Stage Renal Disease (ESRD).**

At this stage, the kidneys cannot clean the blood effectively anymore. Dialysis becomes a life-support treatment.

**Dialysis Options: Hemodialysis (HD) vs Peritoneal Dialysis (PD)**

When doctors say dialysis is needed, families often panic. But understanding the options helps reduce fear.

There are two main types:

**1. Hemodialysis (HD)**

In Hemodialysis:

Blood is taken out of the body through a machine. The machine filters the blood. Clean blood is returned to the body.

This usually happens:

- ✓ *2–3 times per week*
- ✓ *At a dialysis center*
- ✓ *Each session lasts 4–5 hours*

Advantages:

- ✓ Performed by trained staff
- ✓ No need to manage daily exchanges at home

Challenges:

- ✓ Travel to center
- ✓ Long waiting hours
- ✓ Fixed schedule
- ✓ Post-dialysis weakness
- ✓ Needle insertion each time

**2. Peritoneal Dialysis (PD)**

In Peritoneal Dialysis:

The patient's own abdominal lining (peritoneum) acts as the filter.

Dialysis fluid is put into the abdomen through a permanent catheter.

Waste and extra water pass into the fluid.

The used fluid is drained out and replaced with fresh fluid.

This is called an **exchange.**

PD is usually done:

At home Several times a day (CAPD) or At night using a machine (APD)

**Why Some Patients Prefer PD**

Every patient's situation is different. But many choose PD for these reasons:

1. Freedom & Flexibility

PD is done at home. No need to travel to hospital multiple times per week.

2. Gentler on the Body

PD removes waste slowly and continuously.

This often causes:

- ✓ Less blood pressure fluctuation
- ✓ Less fatigue
- ✓ More stable energy levels

3. Fewer Dietary Restrictions (in some cases)

Some patients on PD have slightly more flexibility with fluids compared to HD — but this depends on medical advice.

4. Independence

Patients feel more in control. They can manage treatment around work, family, or travel (with planning).

5. Better for Heart Health (in many cases)

Since fluid removal is gradual, it is often easier on the heart compared to rapid removal in HD.

However, PD requires discipline.
Cleanliness is critical. Infection control is life-saving.
Caregiver involvement is essential.
That is why this guide exists.

**The Emotional Journey of Patients & Families**

Kidney failure does not just affect the body. It affects the mind and emotions.

Common feelings in patients:

- ✓ Fear
- ✓ Anger
- ✓ Sadness
- ✓ Guilt ("I am a burden")
- ✓ Anxiety about infection
- ✓ Frustration with restrictions

Common feelings in caregivers:

- ✓ Shock
- ✓ Overwhelm
- ✓ Fear of making mistakes

- ✓ Sleep disturbance
- ✓ Financial worry
- ✓ Emotional exhaustion

These reactions are normal.

The first few weeks are the hardest. Everything feels complicated. Every step feels scary.

But here is the truth:

With routine and proper training, PD becomes manageable.

Thousands of families successfully perform exchanges every day at home.

Confidence comes with:

- ✓ Understanding
- ✓ Practice
- ✓ Discipline
- ✓ Support

**Important Reminder for Caregivers**

You are not just helping with a medical procedure.

You are:

- ✓ *Protecting against infection*
- ✓ *Monitoring warning signs*
- ✓ *Offering emotional strength*
- ✓ *Maintaining hope*
- ✓ *Your role is powerful.*

But you must also care for yourself:

- ✓ Take breaks
- ✓ Ask for help
- ✓ Stay connected
- ✓ Share responsibilities when possible

A calm caregiver creates a calm patient.

**Closing Thoughts for This Chapter**

Kidney failure is serious — but it is not the end of life.

Peritoneal Dialysis is not just a treatment. It is a structured system that allows patients to continue living — eating, talking, working, loving, laughing.
Understanding what is happening inside the body reduces fear.
In the next chapters, we will move from understanding to action — learning exactly how to perform exchanges safely and confidently.

You are not alone on this journey. And step by step, you will become confident.

# Chapter 2:
# What is Peritoneal Dialysis?

When families first hear the words Peritoneal Dialysis, it can sound complicated and frightening. But when we break it down into simple steps, it becomes much easier to understand.

Peritoneal Dialysis (PD) is a way of cleaning the blood when the kidneys can no longer do their job properly. It is a treatment that happens inside the body, using a natural lining in the abdomen as a filter.

Let us understand this step by step.

**How PD Works – A Simple Explanation**

Think of the body as a house. In a healthy house, waste water goes out through proper drainage pipes. If the drainage system stops working, dirty water begins to collect. That would make the house unsafe.

The kidneys are like the drainage system of the body. When they fail, waste and extra water begin to build up in the blood.

Peritoneal Dialysis works by using a special cleansing fluid and the patient's own abdominal lining to remove that waste.

Here is what happens during PD:

A soft tube called a **catheter** is surgically placed into the patient's abdomen.

A special sterile dialysis fluid is allowed to flow into the abdomen through that tube.

The fluid stays inside for a few hours.

During that time, waste products and extra water move from the blood vessels into the dialysis fluid.

The used fluid is then drained out and replaced with fresh fluid.

This process is called an **exchange**.

It sounds simple — and in many ways, it is. But it must be done carefully and cleanly every single time.

### The Peritoneal Membrane – The Body's Natural Filter

Inside the abdomen, there is a thin lining called the **peritoneum**. This lining covers the abdominal organs. The peritoneum has a rich supply of tiny blood vessels. These blood vessels carry waste-filled blood.

The dialysis fluid that we put into the abdomen comes into contact with this lining. Through a natural process (like a sponge drawing water), waste and extra fluid pass from the blood vessels into the dialysis fluid.

No machine is needed to filter the blood directly. The body's own membrane acts as the filter.

This is one reason PD feels gentler for many patients — the blood never leaves the body.

### What Happens During an Exchange?

An exchange has three main parts:

**1. Fill**

Fresh dialysis fluid flows into the abdomen.

**2. Dwell**

The fluid stays inside for a few hours. During this time, waste and extra water move into the fluid.

**3. Drain**

The used fluid is drained out into a bag.

Then the cycle repeats.

This continuous cleaning helps maintain a safer balance in the body.

## Types of Peritoneal Dialysis

There are two main types of PD. Both work in the same way. The difference is when and how exchanges are done.

### 1. CAPD (Continuous Ambulatory Peritoneal Dialysis)

This is the most common type. Done manually. Usually 3–4 exchanges per day.

Each exchange takes about 20–30 minutes.

Fluid stays inside for 4-8 hours between exchanges.

It does not require a machine. The patient or caregiver performs the exchanges during the day.

Many patients prefer CAPD because:

- ✓ It is simple.
- ✓ No electricity is required.
- ✓ It allows flexibility in timing.

However, it requires discipline and clean surroundings every time.

### 2. APD (Automated Peritoneal Dialysis)

This uses a machine called a cycler. Done mostly at night while the patient sleeps.

The machine automatically performs several exchanges.

Usually connected for 8–10 hours overnight.

Advantages:

- ✓ Daytime is free.
- ✓ Fewer daytime interruptions.

However:

- ✓ Requires electricity.
- ✓ The machine must be maintained properly.
- ✓ Patients need proper training to use it safely.

Your nephrologist will decide which method is suitable based on:

- ✓ Lifestyle
- ✓ Medical condition
- ✓ Home environment
- ✓ Patient preference

**Advantages of Peritoneal Dialysis**

Many families choose PD because of the following benefits:

1. Home-Based Treatment

No frequent hospital visits for dialysis sessions. This saves travel time and reduces stress.

2. Gentle Fluid Removal

Since dialysis happens continuously, fluid removal is slower and steadier.
This often means:

- ✓ Fewer sudden drops in blood pressure
- ✓ Less dizziness
- ✓ Less exhaustion after exchanges

3. Greater Independence

Patients can plan their day better. Some continue working or managing daily life activities.

4. No Needles Each Session

Unlike hemodialysis, PD does not require needle insertion every time.

5. More Stable Body Chemistry

Because PD is continuous, there are fewer large swings in body waste levels.

**Risks & Responsibilities**

While PD offers freedom, it also comes with serious responsibilities.

The biggest risk in PD is **infection**, especially:

1. Peritonitis (Infection inside the abdomen)

Warning signs:

- ✓ Cloudy drain fluid
- ✓ Abdominal pain
- ✓ Fever
- ✓ Nausea

This requires immediate medical attention.

2. Exit Site Infection

The area where the catheter comes out of the body can get infected if not cleaned properly.

Signs:

- ✓ Redness
- ✓ Swelling
- ✓ Pus
- ✓ Pain

3. Fluid Problems

Too much fluid removed → weakness, dizziness. Too little fluid removed → swelling, breathlessness.

4. Hernia

Increased pressure inside the abdomen can sometimes cause hernia.

5. Catheter Blockage

Improper drainage can occur if catheter position changes.

**Responsibilities of the Caregiver**

Peritoneal Dialysis is safe when done correctly.
But it requires:

- ✓ Strict hand-washing every time
- ✓ Clean environment
- ✓ Checking dialysis solution carefully
- ✓ Watching for changes in drain fluid
- ✓ Monitoring patient symptoms
- ✓ Keeping emergency contact numbers ready

One careless moment can increase infection risk. That may sound frightening — but with routine and discipline, it becomes manageable.

**A Realistic View**

In the beginning: Everything feels difficult.

You will double-check each step. You may feel anxious. That is normal.

After a few weeks:

- ✓ *The routine becomes familiar.*
- ✓ *Your hands move confidently.*
- ✓ *You begin to notice small details.*
- ✓ *You understand your patient's body better.*

Many caregivers say*: "I was scared at first. Now it is part of our life."*

**Final Thoughts**

Peritoneal Dialysis is not just a medical treatment. It is a partnership between:

- ✓ The patient
- ✓ The caregiver
- ✓ The doctor
- ✓ And discipline

When done carefully, PD allows patients to live longer, fuller lives at home.

In the next chapters, we will move from understanding to practical steps — preparing the environment, mastering hand hygiene, and performing exchanges safely.

Knowledge reduces fear. Routine builds confidence. Clean hands save lives.

# PART 2:
# ROLE OF THE CAREGIVER

# Chapter 3:
# The Responsibility of a PD Caregiver

When a person starts Peritoneal Dialysis, life does not change only for the patient. It changes for the whole family — especially for the caregiver.

A PD caregiver is not just someone who "helps." You become the safety guard, the observer, the reminder, the encourager, and sometimes the strength when the patient feels weak.

This chapter is about understanding your responsibility — not to frighten you, but to prepare you. Because when you know your role clearly, you work with confidence.

**Infection Control Is Life-Saving**

Let us say this clearly: In Peritoneal Dialysis, **cleanliness is not optional — it is life-saving.**

The dialysis fluid goes directly into the abdomen. If germs enter during the exchange, they can cause a serious infection called peritonitis. This is not a small problem. It can require hospitalization and can even be dangerous.

That is why hand-washing, masking, cleaning the table, checking the solution — all these steps are not just "procedures." They are protection.

As a caregiver, your most important duty is infection prevention.

This means:

- ✓ *Washing hands properly every single time*
- ✓ *Not rushing the process*
- ✓ *Wearing a mask during exchanges*
- ✓ *Keeping pets away from the procedure area*

- ✓ *Avoiding fans or open windows during exchanges*
- ✓ *Never touching connection points unnecessarily*
- ✓ *Checking that the dialysis fluid is clear and not expired*

Even on days when you feel tired.
Even on days when you are in a hurry.
Discipline in hygiene protects the patient's life.

**Mental & Emotional Support**

Kidney failure affects the mind just as much as the body. Patients may not always say it openly, but they often feel:

- ✓ *Fear of infection*
- ✓ *Fear of becoming dependent*
- ✓ *Fear of financial burden*
- ✓ *Sadness about lifestyle changes*
- ✓ *Anger about restrictions*

Sometimes they may become irritable. Sometimes quiet. Sometimes withdrawn.

As a caregiver, your emotional presence matters more than perfect words.

Simple things help:

*Sit with them during exchanges.*
*Talk normally — not always about illness.*
*Encourage them gently.*
*Avoid scolding or blaming.*
*Celebrate small improvements.*

Never say: *"You are a burden."*

Instead say: *"We are managing this together."*

Also remember: caregivers also feel tired and stressed. It is okay to feel overwhelmed. You are human.

If you feel emotionally exhausted:

- ✓ Share responsibilities when possible.
- ✓ Talk to another family member.
- ✓ Speak to the doctor if you feel anxious.
- ✓ Take short breaks.

A calm caregiver creates a calm patient.

**Discipline & Routine**

Peritoneal Dialysis works best when it becomes a habit.

- ✓ Same place.
- ✓ Same steps.
- ✓ Same order.
- ✓ Routine reduces mistakes.

Create a fixed exchange area in the home. Do not change it often.

Create fixed exchange timings. Try not to delay unless absolutely necessary.

Before each exchange:

- ✓ Check the supplies.
- ✓ Check the solution strength.
- ✓ Check expiry.
- ✓ Check clarity.
- ✓ Check cleanliness of the area.

Do not skip steps because "everything looks fine."

Routine builds safety.

Over time, you will notice something important — when you follow a disciplined routine, the patient feels more secure. They trust the process more.

**Documentation Habit**

This is a very important but often ignored responsibility.

Write things down.

Maintain a small notebook or printed log sheet where you record:

- ✓ Date and time of exchange
- ✓ Type and strength of solution used
- ✓ Drain volume
- ✓ Inflow volume
- ✓ Appearance of drain fluid (clear, cloudy, blood-tinged)
- ✓ Patient complaints (pain, dizziness, fever)
- ✓ Blood pressure (if monitored)
- ✓ Weight (daily, preferably at the same time)

Why is this important?

Because small changes over days tell a story. A doctor can help much better when you give accurate information. For example: Instead of saying, *"Urine is less,"*

you can say, *"For the past 3 days, urine output has reduced from 500 ml to 300 ml."*

Instead of saying, *"Fluid looks different,"* you can say, *"Since yesterday evening, the drain fluid is slightly cloudy."*

Documentation reduces guesswork.

It also reduces panic because you can see patterns clearly.

**Common Caregiver Mistakes**

Even careful caregivers can make mistakes. Being aware helps you avoid them.

1. Rushing the Procedure

Hurrying increases contamination risk. Always allow enough time.

2. Touching Sterile Points

The catheter tip and connection points must not be touched unnecessarily.

3. Ignoring Slight Cloudiness

Even mild cloudiness must be taken seriously. Early action prevents serious infection.

4. Skipping Hand-washing Steps
Quick rinse is not enough. Follow the full hand-washing method.
5. Not Checking Expiry or Strength
Using the wrong solution strength can cause fluid imbalance.
6. Becoming Overconfident
After months of smooth exchanges, some caregivers become relaxed about discipline. That is when mistakes happen.
7. Ignoring Personal Health
If you are sick (fever, cough, infection), take extra precautions. Wear a proper mask and consider asking another trained person to assist if needed.

**You Are Part of the Treatment**

Many caregivers underestimate their importance.
The doctor prescribes treatment. The dialysis fluid works inside the body. But the caregiver ensures the treatment happens safely every day.
Your role is active, not passive.
You are:

- ✓ *The infection barrier*
- ✓ *The daily monitor*
- ✓ *The routine manager*
- ✓ *The emotional anchor*

That is a powerful responsibility.

**Final Words for This Chapter**

Do not aim to be perfect. Aim to be careful. Do not aim to be fearless. Aim to be disciplined. You will learn. You will grow confident. You will make this routine part of life.

***Peritoneal Dialysis is not managed by medicine alone. It is managed by careful hands and steady hearts.***

# Chapter 4:
# Preparing the Home Environment

**Clean Space. Safe Exchange. Peace of Mind.**

Peritoneal Dialysis does not require a hospital room — but it does require a clean, organized space.

Many caregivers ask:

*"Does my house need to be perfect?"* The answer is no.

It does not need to be perfect. But it must be **clean, controlled, and consistent.**

In PD, germs are the biggest enemy. And most infections do not happen because of the dialysis fluid — they happen because of contamination during setup.

This chapter will help you prepare your home in a practical and realistic way.

**Clean Designated Exchange Area**

The first rule:

Choose <u>one fixed place</u> for exchanges.

Do not keep changing rooms.

It can be:

- ✓ A bedroom corner
- ✓ A clean section of the living room
- ✓ A small study area

But once chosen, it should become your PD zone.

**Why a Fixed Area?**

When you use the same place every time:

- ✓ *You reduce confusion.*
- ✓ *You reduce mistakes.*
- ✓ *You maintain better cleanliness.*
- ✓ *You build routine.*

**What That Area Should Have:**

- ✓ A small table or tray for supplies
- ✓ Enough space to hang the PD solution bag
- ✓ A clean floor area (for drain collection if required)
- ✓ Good lighting
- ✓ Minimal movement around

Before every exchange:

- ✓ Wipe the table with gauze and sanitizer.
- ✓ Clean the PD stand.
- ✓ Clean the solution bag surface.
- ✓ Ensure the area is free from clutter.
- ✓ Do not use the exchange table for eating, ironing, or other daily work.

That table is only for PD.

**Ventilation & Lighting**

The room should be well-lit so you can clearly see:

- ✓ Connection points
- ✓ Fluid clarity
- ✓ Cap closures
- ✓ Clamp positions

Poor lighting increases small errors. Natural light is good. But avoid strong air flow from open windows during the procedure.

**Ventilation Guidelines:**

- ✓ Room should not feel suffocating.
- ✓ Windows can be opened before preparation.
- ✓ Close windows during the exchange if there is dust outside.
- ✓ Avoid strong cross-ventilation during connections.
- ✓ Fresh air is good. Dust movement is not.

**Avoiding Fans & Dust During Exchange**

This is very important.

When the connection between catheter and solution is open, it is a critical moment. Even tiny airborne particles can carry germs.

Before starting:

- ✓ Switch off ceiling fans.
- ✓ Switch off pedestal fans.
- ✓ Turn off air coolers.
- ✓ Avoid direct air from AC blowing on the exchange area. (best- if AC is off)

If the weather is hot:

- ✓ Cool the room first.
- ✓ Then switch off airflow just before starting connections.

Also:

- ✓ Do not sweep or dust the room just before exchange.
- ✓ Do not shake bedsheets nearby.
- ✓ Avoid walking in and out during connection time.
- ✓ Keep movement minimal.

**Lever-Type Taps (Important from SOP)**

After washing hands properly, your hands must not touch contaminated surfaces again.

If you wash hands and then turn off the tap with your fingers, you may re-contaminate them.

That is why **lever-type taps are recommended.**

With lever taps:

- ✓ You can push them down using your elbow.
- ✓ You do not need to touch with fingers.

If lever taps are not available:

- ✓ Use a clean tissue to close the tap.
- ✓ Do not use your washed hands directly.

After drying:

- ✓ Use hand sanitizer again before touching supplies.
- ✓ Hand hygiene is not one step — it is continuous awareness.

**Keeping Pets Away**

Pets are family members. But during PD exchanges, they must stay away.

Animals carry bacteria on:

- ✓ Fur
- ✓ Paws
- ✓ Saliva

Even if they look clean, microscopic germs can cause infection.

Before exchange:

- ✓ Keep pets in another room.
- ✓ Close the door.
- ✓ Do not allow them to jump onto the exchange table.
- ✓ Do not allow them near dialysis supplies.
- ✓ After the exchange is complete and everything is sealed properly, normal interaction can resume, though better not to have them around the patient

During exchange time, the room must be a controlled environment.

**Creating a PD Station**

A PD station means organizing all supplies in one dedicated place.

This helps in:

- ✓ Reducing last-minute searching
- ✓ Preventing contamination
- ✓ Saving time

- ✓ Avoiding panic

**What Your PD Station Should Include:**

**For Exchange:**

- ✓ PD solution bags (organized by strength)
- ✓ Mini caps
- ✓ Blue clamps
- ✓ Gloves
- ✓ Masks
- ✓ Hand sanitizer
- ✓ Liquid soap
- ✓ Clean gauze
- ✓ Waste disposal bag
- ✓ Newspaper sheets (as per your SOP — one for waste, one for drain fluid if needed)

**For Dressing Care:**

- ✓ Gauze
- ✓ Ointment
- ✓ Benzodine (or prescribed cleaning solution)
- ✓ Transparent tape
- ✓ Microtape
- ✓ Scissors (clean and reserved only for PD use)

Keep these items:

- ✓ In closed storage
- ✓ Away from moisture
- ✓ Away from children
- ✓ Away from kitchen area

Check stock regularly.
Do not wait until the last bag is finished.

**Organizing PD Solutions**

Store PD solution bags:

- ✓ In a clean cupboard or shelf
- ✓ Away from direct sunlight
- ✓ At normal room temperature
- ✓ Off the floor (preferably on a rack)

Before each use:

- ✓ Check expiry date
- ✓ Check strength (2.5%, 7.5%, or as prescribed)
- ✓ Check for leaks
- ✓ Check clarity (no cloudiness)

Never use a damaged bag.

**Personal Preparation Before Starting**

Before entering the PD zone:

- ✓ Tie hair back.
- ✓ Remove watches, rings, bracelets.
- ✓ Trim nails short.
- ✓ Wear clean clothes.
- ✓ Wear a mask.

Simple steps reduce contamination risk.

**Limiting Room Traffic**

During exchange:

- ✓ Only the caregiver (and patient) should be present.
- ✓ No visitors.
- ✓ No children running in and out.
- ✓ No phone handling during connection stage.

If you must take a phone call:

- ✓ Complete the connection first.
- ✓ Sanitize hands again before touching supplies.

**Making the Environment Calm**

A calm space helps both caregiver and patient.

Avoid loud TV. Avoid arguments. Keep the atmosphere steady.

When the patient feels relaxed:

- ✓ Blood pressure stays stable.
- ✓ Procedure goes smoothly.

**Final Thoughts**

Preparing the home environment is not about luxury. It is about control. You cannot control everything in kidney disease.

But you can control:

- ✓ Clean hands
- ✓ Clean space
- ✓ Clean supplies
- ✓ Calm routine

That control protects the patient every single day.

# PART 3:
# INFECTION CONTROL – FOUNDATION OF SAFETY

# Chapter 5:
# The 6-Step Clinical Hand-washing Technique

Clean Hands Save Lives

If there is one habit that protects a Peritoneal Dialysis patient more than anything else, it is proper handwashing.

- ✓ Not quick washing.
- ✓ Not rinsing.
- ✓ Not "just sanitizer."
- ✓ Proper, structured, clinical handwashing.

Many infections in PD do not happen because something major went wrong. They happen because of one small shortcut — a rushed wash, an unclean thumb, or touching something after washing.

This chapter will teach you exactly how to wash your hands correctly — and why every single movement matters.

**Before You Begin**

Before washing:

- ✓ *Remove rings, bangles, bracelets, and watches.*
- ✓ *Keep nails short and clean.*
- ✓ *Do not wear artificial nails or nail polish during exchanges.*
- ✓ *Tie back long hair.*
- ✓ *Wear clean clothes.*

Now you are ready.

**The 6-Step Clinical Handwashing Technique**

- ✓ Use clean running water and liquid soap.

- ✓ Rub hands for at least 40–60 seconds.
- ✓ Do not rush.

**Step 1: Palm to Palm**

Rub your palms together with soap.

Move them in circular motion. Create foam. Cover the entire palm surface.

Why This Matters

- ✓ Your palms touch everything — bags, clamps, table surfaces. Germs often sit here. This first step removes surface dirt and bacteria.
- ✓ Do not wash only fingertips. Cover the full palm.

**Step 2: Right Palm Over Left Hand (Back of Hand) and Vice Versa**

Place your right palm over the back of your left hand.

Interlock fingers slightly and rub.

Then switch sides.

Why This Matters

- ✓ The back of the hand is often ignored. But it touches clothing, tables, and doors.
- ✓ Germs hide here easily because people forget to clean it properly.

**Step 3: Palm to Palm with Fingers Interlaced**

Join your hands palm to palm again — but this time interlock your fingers and rub.

Move back and forth.

Why This Matters

- ✓ Between fingers is a common hiding place for bacteria. Sweat and moisture collect here.
- ✓ If this area is missed, germs can transfer during connection handling.

**Step 4: Back of Fingers to Opposing Palm**

Bend your fingers and rub the backs of them against your opposite palm.

Do both hands.

Why This Matters

- ✓ The knuckle area and backs of fingers often escape cleaning.
- ✓ These areas frequently touch sterile caps and tubes during exchange.

**Step 5: Rotational Rubbing of Thumbs**

Hold your left thumb in your right palm and rotate it firmly.

Then switch.

Why This Matters

- ✓ The thumb is the most used finger.
- ✓ It grips clamps. It adjusts caps. It steadies tubes.
- ✓ But it is also the most neglected in washing.
- ✓ Many people forget to clean the thumb properly.

**Step 6: Fingertips & Nails in Opposite Palm**

Rub fingertips of one hand in circular motion against the opposite palm.

Then switch.

Why This Matters

- ✓ Under the nails and fingertips carry the highest number of germs.
- ✓ When connecting PD tubes, fingertips come very close to sterile openings.
- ✓ If this step is skipped, infection risk increases significantly.

**Rinse Properly**

After completing all six steps:

- ✓ Rinse hands thoroughly under running water.
- ✓ Keep fingertips pointing downward.
- ✓ Let water flow from wrist to fingertips.
- ✓ Do not let dirty water flow back from wrist to fingers.

**Drying Hands**

- ✓ Use clean disposable paper towel.
- ✓ Dry completely.
- ✓ Do not use shared cloth towels.
- ✓ Wet hands attract bacteria faster.

**Closing the Tap**

If you have a lever-type tap (though very much recommended):

Push it down with your elbow.

If not:

Use a paper towel to close it.

Do not touch tap directly with clean fingers.

**When to Repeat Handwashing**

Repeat full handwashing:

- ✓ Before every exchange.
- ✓ Before exit-site dressing.
- ✓ After using the toilet.
- ✓ After coughing or sneezing.
- ✓ After touching pets.
- ✓ After touching phone or door handles during procedure.
- ✓ If you accidentally touch a non-sterile surface.
- ✓ If in doubt — wash again.
- ✓ It is better to wash twice than regret once.

**When to Use Hand Sanitizer**

Sanitizer is an extra protection — not a replacement.

Use sanitizer:

- ✓ After drying hands, before touching PD supplies.
- ✓ If you accidentally touch something during setup.

After removing gloves.

Between minor handling steps if required.
Remember:
If hands are visibly dirty, sanitizer is not enough. You must wash with soap and water first.

**Common Hygiene Errors**

Even experienced caregivers sometimes make these mistakes.
Be aware of them.
1. Washing Too Fast
Rushing through steps reduces effectiveness.
Handwashing should take at least 40 seconds.
2. Missing Thumbs or Fingertips
These are the most commonly skipped areas.
3. Wearing Rings or Bangles
Germs hide under jewelry.
Remove them before washing.
4. Turning Off Tap with Clean Hands
This re-contaminates hands.
Always use elbow or tissue.
5. Touching Phone After Washing
Mobile phones carry heavy bacteria.
If touched, sanitize again.
6. Long or Artificial Nails
These trap bacteria and increase infection risk.
Keep nails short and simple.
7. Skipping Mask
Handwashing is not enough. During connection, always wear a mask.
Breathing or talking directly over open connections increases contamination risk.

**Why Handwashing Is the Foundation**

Peritoneal Dialysis is done at home.

There is no hospital infection control team standing next to you.
You are the infection control team.
One proper wash can prevent:

- ✓ Peritonitis
- ✓ Hospital admission
- ✓ IV antibiotics
- ✓ Severe complications

It may feel repetitive. It may feel strict. But it protects the patient every single day.

**Final Thoughts**

Never underestimate your hands.

- ✓ They connect the tubing.
- ✓ They open the caps.
- ✓ They protect the abdomen.

Clean hands are not just hygiene.
They are safety. They are discipline. They are life-saving.

# Chapter 6:
# Setting Up for the Procedure (Pre-Exchange Preparation)

**Preparation Prevents Problems**

In Peritoneal Dialysis, the exchange itself is only half the job. The other half — and equally important — is preparation.

Many infections happen not during draining or filling, but during poor setup. If you prepare properly, the exchange becomes smooth and safe.

This chapter will guide you step-by-step exactly how to prepare before every exchange. Do not skip this stage. Good preparation builds confidence.

**Step 1: Gather All Required Items First**

Never start washing hands and then search for supplies.

Before you begin:

- ✓ Check everything is available.
- ✓ Arrange it neatly.
- ✓ Make sure nothing is missing.

There are two categories of items:

- ✓ *Dressing Items*
- ✓ *Exchange Items*

Keep them stored separately but organized.

**Dressing Items Checklist**

(For Exit Site Care)

Keep these ready when doing dressing:

- ✓ Gauze
- ✓ Hand sanitizer
- ✓ Ointment (as prescribed)
- ✓ Scissors (clean and reserved only for PD use)

- ✓ Blue sheet (clean surface cover)
- ✓ Benzodine or prescribed cleaning solution
- ✓ Gloves
- ✓ Mask
- ✓ Microtape
- ✓ Transparent tape

Important:
Scissors must not be used for household purposes.
Dressing materials must be stored in a clean, dry place.
Check expiry of ointments regularly.

**Exchange Items Checklist**

(For PD Fluid Exchange)
Keep the following ready:

- ✓ Liquid handwash soap
- ✓ Table or tray for arranging items
- ✓ PD solution stand (for hanging bag)
- ✓ PD solution bag (correct strength)
- ✓ Blue sheet
- ✓ Mini cap
- ✓ Blue clamp
- ✓ Hand sanitizer
- ✓ Gloves
- ✓ Mask
- ✓ Newspaper sheets (2 pieces)

Arrange these neatly before washing hands.
Do not open any sterile packaging until instructed in the exchange steps.

**Step 2: Checking the PD Solution**

Before every exchange, carefully inspect the PD solution bag.
Never assume it is correct.
1. Check the Right Strength

PD solution comes in different strengths (for example 2.5% and 7.5%).
Your doctor will prescribe which strength to use and at what time.
Generally:
2.5 strength – commonly used for 6 to 8 hours dwell
7.5 strength – may be used for longer dwell (around 12 hours) depending on medical advice
Using the wrong strength can cause:

- ✓ Too much fluid removal → weakness, low BP
- ✓ Too little fluid removal → swelling, breathlessness

Always double-check the label before opening.
2. Check Expiry Date
Look carefully at the expiry date printed on the bag.
Never use an expired bag — even if it expired yesterday.
Expired solution may not be sterile or effective.
3. Check for Leaks
Gently squeeze the bag.
Look for:

- ✓ Wetness on outer cover
- ✓ Cracks
- ✓ Tears

If there is any leak — discard the bag.
4. Check for Cloudiness
Hold the bag up to light.
The solution must be completely clear.
If it looks cloudy or has particles:
Do not use it. Inform your supplier or doctor.
Clarity is essential.

**Step 3: Preparing the Table Area**
Now prepare your exchange space carefully.
Table Setup Procedure

- ✓ Clean the table or tray with gauze and sanitizer.
- ✓ Allow it to dry.
- ✓ Wipe the PD stand with sanitizer.
- ✓ Clean the outer surface of the PD solution bag.
- ✓ Place items in organized order.
- ✓ Arrange items so you do not have to cross your hands over sterile parts.
- ✓ Keep sterile and non-sterile items separate.
- ✓ Do not place items directly on the bare floor.

**Step 4: Newspaper Placement System**

This is a simple but practical system.

Place two newspapers on the floor:

- ✓ One for waste disposal
- ✓ One under the drain bag (if required)

Why?

- ✓ It prevents fluid from spilling on the floor.
- ✓ It keeps waste organized.
- ✓ It reduces contamination risk.

After exchange:

- ✓ Fold newspapers carefully.
- ✓ Dispose properly.
- ✓ Never leave used drain bags open in the room.

**Step 5: Handwashing Before Touching Supplies**

Now perform the full 6-step handwash method.

After drying:

- ✓ Close tap using elbow or tissue.
- ✓ Sanitize hands again.
- ✓ Wear mask.
- ✓ Wear gloves (if required for specific steps).

- ✓ Do not start setting up connections before proper hygiene.

**Step 6: Sanitizing Items Individually**

This is often overlooked.

Before placing items on table:

- ✓ Wipe each item with gauze and sanitizer.
- ✓ Wipe PD stand.
- ✓ Wipe bag surface.
- ✓ Wipe clamps.
- ✓ Do not soak items — just clean outer surfaces.

This reduces the chance of outside contamination.

Remember:

*Outer surfaces may have been handled during packing or transport.*

**Step 7: Wearing PPE (Personal Protective Equipment)**

Always wear:

- ✓ Mask
- ✓ Gloves (when handling connection points or dressing)

Mask is essential during connection and disconnection.

Talking or breathing directly over open catheter ends can introduce germs.

If caregiver has:

- ✓ Cold
- ✓ Cough
- ✓ Fever

Extra caution is required.

Avoid performing exchange if you are unwell, if possible. If unavoidable, wear mask properly and maintain strict hygiene.

**Final Pre-Exchange Check**

Before beginning drain:

Ask yourself:

- ✓ *Is the room calm?*
- ✓ *Is the fan switched off?*
- ✓ *Are pets away?*
- ✓ *Are all items ready?*
- ✓ *Is the solution checked?*
- ✓ *Are hands washed?*
- ✓ *Is mask worn?*

If all answers are yes — proceed.

If unsure — stop and correct first.

Never rush.

**Why Preparation Is So Important**

Preparation may feel repetitive.

But it prevents:

- ✓ Infection
- ✓ Wrong solution use
- ✓ Panic during exchange
- ✓ Forgotten steps
- ✓ Emergency situations

When preparation becomes habit, the exchange becomes smooth.

**Final Thoughts**

Setting up properly is a sign of responsible caregiving.

It shows respect for the process.

It protects the patient.

It protects your effort.

Good preparation reduces fear.

And when preparation is disciplined, Peritoneal Dialysis becomes manageable and safe at home.

# PART 4:
# THE PERITONEAL DIALYSIS EXCHANGE – STEP-BY-STEP SOP

# Chapter 7:
# Drain Phase (Outflow Procedure)

**The First Step of Every Exchange**

The drain phase is the beginning of every PD exchange.

This is the stage where the used dialysis fluid — the fluid that has collected waste and extra water from the body — is removed.

Never rush this part.

The drain phase tells you important information about the patient's condition. It also prepares the abdomen for fresh fluid.

Take your time. Stay calm. Follow the same order every time.

**Before You Begin the Drain**

Confirm:

- ✓ *Hands are washed using the full 6-step method.*
- ✓ *Mask is worn properly.*
- ✓ *Table and items are sanitized.*
- ✓ *Correct PD solution bag is ready and checked.*
- ✓ *Newspapers are placed.*
- ✓ *Fan is switched off.*
- ✓ *Patient is seated comfortably.*
- ✓ *The patient should sit upright or slightly reclined. Good posture helps drainage.*

Now you are ready to begin.

**Step 1: Loosen the Bottom White Mini Cap**

At the end of the patient's catheter, there will be a protective white mini cap.

This cap protects the internal catheter from contamination between exchanges.

Carefully:

- ✓ Hold the catheter steady.
- ✓ Gently loosen the bottom white mini cap.
- ✓ Do not touch the open connection tip.
- ✓ Keep movements controlled and clean.
- ✓ Do not let the open end swing freely.

This is a sterile area. Treat it with respect.

**Step 2: Pull Green Connector from the PD Solution Bag & Connect to Bottom**

From the PD solution bag, locate the green connector tubing.

Carefully:

- ✓ Remove the protective cover from the green connector.
- ✓ Without touching the connecting ends directly,
- ✓ Connect the green tubing to the patient's catheter.
- ✓ Make sure it fits securely.
- ✓ Do not force it.

Once connected properly, you are ready to allow drainage.

**Step 3: Open the White Top Cap**

Now:

- ✓ Open the white top cap as instructed in your training.
- ✓ Ensure clamps are positioned correctly.
- ✓ Once opened properly, gravity will begin the drain.

**Step 4: The Drain Process Explained**

Now the used dialysis fluid will begin flowing out from the patient's abdomen into the drain bag.

You will see fluid moving through the tubing.

This fluid has:

- ✓ Waste products
- ✓ Extra water
- ✓ Toxins removed from the blood

It should flow smoothly.

**What Normal Drain Looks Like**

The outflow fluid should be:

- ✓ Clear
- ✓ Light yellow or straw colored
- ✓ Without particles

A useful home check:

If you place the drain bag over newspaper, you should be able to see the letters clearly through the fluid.

Clear fluid usually means no infection.

**What to Watch During Drain**

Stay present during this phase.

Observe:

- ✓ Is fluid flowing steadily?
- ✓ Is patient comfortable?
- ✓ Is there pain?
- ✓ Mild pulling sensation can be normal.
- ✓ Severe pain is not normal.

If patient feels strong pain:

- ✓ Check tube position.
- ✓ Ensure there is no kink.
- ✓ Slightly change patient position.

If problem continues — contact doctor.

**Abnormal Signs (Very Important)**

During drain, look carefully.

1. Cloudy Fluid

If the fluid looks cloudy or milky:

This may be a sign of infection (peritonitis).

Contact your nephrologist immediately.

Do not ignore even slight cloudiness.

**2. Blood in Fluid**

If fluid looks red or pink:

Inform doctor immediately.

Sometimes slight pink color may happen after catheter movement, but it must always be reported.

**3. White Rice-Like Particles (Fibrin)**

If you see small white string-like or rice-like particles:

These are called fibrin.

Your doctor may advise adding heparin injection to the PD solution.

Do not self-medicate without instruction.

Always inform your nephrologist.

**Time Expectations**

Drain time varies.

Usually: 10 to 20 minutes

Sometimes slightly longer

It depends on:

- ✓ Patient position
- ✓ Catheter placement
- ✓ Amount of fluid
- ✓ Body condition

Do not rush the drain.

Let gravity do the work.

If drainage is slow:

Ask patient to change position slightly.

Ask patient to cough gently.

Check tubing for kinks.

Never squeeze the abdomen forcefully.

**Complete Drain Is Important**

Allow as much fluid as possible to drain.

Incomplete drainage can:

- ✓ Reduce dialysis effectiveness
- ✓ Cause discomfort during inflow
- ✓ Increase fluid overload risk

However, do not panic if small residual amount remains.

Follow your doctor's guidance.

**Stay Calm During Drain**

Drain phase is not just mechanical.

It is also observation time.

Use this time to:

- ✓ *Ask patient how they feel.*
- ✓ *Observe facial expression.*
- ✓ *Check for abdominal tenderness.*
- ✓ *Notice energy level.*

Small changes noticed early prevent bigger problems.

**Once Drain Is Complete**

When fluid stops flowing:

- ✓ Ensure drain bag contains expected volume.
- ✓ Check color and clarity one more time.
- ✓ Close clamps as instructed before moving to inflow stage.
- ✓ Do not disconnect casually.
- ✓ Follow sequence strictly.

**Common Mistakes During Drain Phase**

Avoid these errors:

- ✓ Touching connection points unnecessarily
- ✓ Talking directly over open catheter
- ✓ Letting tubing touch unclean surfaces
- ✓ Rushing to start inflow before drain is complete
- ✓ Ignoring mild cloudiness
- ✓ Not checking drain amount
- ✓ Discipline during drain prevents complications.

**Emotional Side of Drain Phase**

Sometimes patients feel tired or frustrated during daily exchanges.

Use this time gently.

Encourage.

Speak calmly.

Do not show anxiety — even if you feel it.
Your steady behavior reassures them.

**Final Thoughts**

The drain phase removes yesterday's waste.
It prepares the body for fresh solution.
It also gives you important health information.
When done calmly and carefully, it becomes routine.
In the next chapter, we will discuss what to monitor closely in the drain fluid and when to contact the doctor immediately.
Careful observation during drain protects the patient every single day.

# Chapter 8: Monitoring the Drain Fluid – Critical Warning Signs

**What the Fluid Is Telling You**

During every PD exchange, the drain phase is not just about removing old fluid.

It is also your daily health check.

The drained fluid gives you important clues about what is happening inside the abdomen. If you learn to observe it carefully, you can catch problems early — before they become serious.

This chapter will teach you exactly what to look for, what is normal, and what requires immediate medical attention.

**The Most Important Rule**

- *Never ignore changes in the drain fluid.*
- *Even small differences matter.*
- *If you are unsure — call the doctor.*
- *It is always better to ask early than regret later.*

**1. Clear Fluid Check**
**(The Newspaper Visibility Test)**

After the fluid has drained into the bag, hold the bag up against light.

The used dialysis fluid should look:

- ✓ Clear
- ✓ Light yellow or straw colored
- ✓ Free of particles

One simple home test is the newspaper test:

- ✓ Place the drain bag over printed newspaper.

- ✓ If you can clearly read the letters through the fluid, it is usually a good sign.
- ✓ Clear fluid generally means there is no infection.

However, always observe carefully. Do not assume.

**2. Cloudy Fluid – Call Doctor Immediately**

If the fluid looks:

- ✓ Milky
- ✓ Foggy
- ✓ Hazy
- ✓ Not transparent

This is a warning sign.

Cloudy fluid is often the earliest sign of **peritonitis**, which is infection inside the abdomen.

- ✓ Do not wait for pain.
- ✓ Do not wait for fever.
- ✓ Cloudy fluid alone is enough reason to contact your nephrologist immediately.
- ✓ The earlier treatment starts, the better the outcome.

Sometimes patients say, *"It looks only slightly cloudy."*

Even slight cloudiness must be reported.

**3. Blood in Outflow – Inform Doctor Immediately**

If the drained fluid appears:

- ✓ Pink
- ✓ Light red
- ✓ Dark red
- ✓ You must inform the doctor.

Sometimes very mild pink color can occur after catheter movement or strain. But it should never be ignored.

Heavy red color or blood clots require urgent attention.

Always note:

- ✓ When it started
- ✓ Whether patient has pain
- ✓ Whether patient had recent constipation or strain

But do not try to diagnose on your own.
Call the doctor.

**4. Fibrin – White Rice-Like Particles**

Sometimes you may see:
*Small white string-like pieces*
*Tiny rice-like particles*
*Soft white threads*
*These are called **fibrin**.*

Fibrin is a protein that can form inside the abdomen and appear in the drain fluid.

It may cause:

- ✓ Slow drainage
- ✓ Tube blockage

This is not always an emergency, but it must be reported.

Doctors often advise adding **heparin** to the PD solution to prevent clotting.

Never add heparin unless your doctor has instructed you clearly on:

- ✓ The dose
- ✓ The method

Follow instructions carefully.
If fibrin appears repeatedly, inform your nephrologist.

**Signs of Peritonitis**

(Infection Inside the Abdomen)
Peritonitis is the most serious infection risk in PD.
Early detection saves lives.
Watch for these signs:

**1. Cloudy Drain Fluid**

This is often the first sign.

**2. Abdominal Pain**

- ✓ Pain may be:
- ✓ Dull
- ✓ Sharp
- ✓ Cramping
- ✓ Continuous

Pain during inflow or drain can be a warning sign.

**3. Fever**

Temperature above normal is concerning.

**4. Nausea or Vomiting**

Some patients feel sick or lose appetite.

**5. Weakness or Fatigue**

Patient may feel unusually tired.

**6. Swelling or Tenderness**

The abdomen may feel sensitive to touch.

If you notice:

- ✓ Cloudy fluid + pain + fever

This is likely peritonitis.

Do not delay. Call the doctor immediately.

**What To Do If You Suspect Infection**

- ✓ Stay calm.
- ✓ Do not panic.
- ✓ Do not stop dialysis unless doctor instructs.
- ✓ Inform your nephrologist immediately.
- ✓ Keep the drain bag available (doctor may ask to see it).
- ✓ Follow medical advice.
- ✓ Early treatment usually involves antibiotics, often given directly into the dialysis fluid.
- ✓ The sooner treatment begins, the better the recovery.

**Other Things to Monitor**

Apart from color and particles, also observe:

**Drain Volume**

If drain amount is much less than usual:

- ✓ There may be blockage.
- ✓ There may be catheter position change.

If drain amount is much more than usual:

- ✓ It may indicate fluid imbalance.

Record volumes daily.

**Odor**

- ✓ Normal drain fluid has very mild or no smell.
- ✓ Strong foul smell may indicate infection.

Report it.

**Trust Your Observation**

You perform exchanges daily.

You know what "normal" looks like for your patient.

If something feels different:

- ✓ Fluid looks slightly unusual
- ✓ Patient feels slightly off
- ✓ Drain pattern changes
- ✓ Do not ignore your instinct.

You are the first line of detection.

**Common Mistakes to Avoid**

- ✓ *Ignoring mild cloudiness*
- ✓ *Assuming pink fluid is normal*
- ✓ *Throwing away drain bag before checking*
- ✓ *Forgetting to record changes*
- ✓ *Waiting overnight to call doctor*

When it comes to infection, time matters.

**Reassurance for Caregivers**

Seeing abnormal fluid can be frightening.

But remember:

- ✓ Many complications are treatable.
- ✓ Early reporting prevents serious problems.

- ✓ You are not expected to diagnose — only to observe and report.

*Observation is your responsibility.*
*Treatment is the doctor's responsibility.*

**Final Thoughts**

Every exchange gives you information.

- ✓ Clear fluid brings relief.
- ✓ Cloudy fluid demands action.
- ✓ Blood demands attention.
- ✓ Fibrin requires guidance.

Your eyes protect the patient.
*Stay observant.*
*Stay disciplined.*
*Stay calm.*

# Chapter 9:
# Inflow Phase (Filling Procedure)

**Refilling the Abdomen Safely and Calmly**

Once the drain phase is complete and the used fluid has been removed, the next step is the inflow phase — filling the abdomen with fresh dialysis solution.

This stage may look simple, but it must be done carefully and in the correct order.

The inflow phase prepares the body for the next few hours of dialysis. If done properly, it should feel smooth and controlled. If rushed or done incorrectly, it can cause discomfort.

Take your time. Follow the same order every day.

Routine builds safety.

**Before Starting Inflow**

Confirm:

- ✓ Drain has completely finished.
- ✓ Drain fluid has been checked for clarity.
- ✓ Abnormal signs (if any) have been noted.
- ✓ Tubing is not twisted.
- ✓ Patient is sitting comfortably.

The patient can remain seated upright or slightly reclined. Good posture helps smooth filling.

**Step 1: Close Caps Correctly**

After the drain is complete:

- ✓ Close the white top cap as instructed.
- ✓ Close the white drain cap properly.
- ✓ Make sure caps are secure but not over-tightened.
- ✓ Do not touch sterile connection points.

This step ensures that the system is properly controlled before beginning inflow.

Always double-check before proceeding.
Small carelessness here can lead to contamination.

**Step 2: Break the Green Tube Twice**

Now locate the green tube that connects to the fresh PD solution bag.
As per your SOP:

- ✓ Break the green tube seal once.
- ✓ Then break it a second time as instructed.

This allows the fresh dialysis fluid to flow when the clamp is opened.
Be gentle but firm.
Make sure the tube is fully broken as required — incomplete breaking may restrict flow.
Do not twist or damage the tubing.

**Step 3: White Clamp Timing (3 Seconds)**

Now comes a small but important step.
Open the white clamp for about **3 seconds**.
Then close it again.
This brief opening allows initial flow adjustment and pressure balance.
It prepares the line for smooth filling.
Count slowly: "One… two… three."
Then close.
Do not rush this part.
It helps prevent sudden pressure during full inflow.

**Step 4: Begin Controlled Inflow**

Now:

- ✓ Open the white top cap as instructed.
- ✓ Open the clamp to allow fresh solution to flow into the abdomen.

The fluid should begin flowing gently.
You will see fluid moving through the tubing.
This is fresh sterile dialysis solution entering the abdominal cavity.

**What Normal Inflow Feels Like**

Most patients feel:

- ✓ Mild fullness
- ✓ Slight cool sensation (if solution is room temperature)
- ✓ Gentle stretching feeling

This is normal.

The inflow should not cause severe pain.

**Monitoring During Inflow**

Stay with the patient.

Observe:

- ✓ Facial expression
- ✓ Body language
- ✓ Breathing pattern

Ask gently:

*"Are you comfortable?"*

**If There Is Mild Discomfort**

Sometimes patients feel:

- ✓ Tightness
- ✓ Mild pressure
- ✓ Slight cramping

You can:

- ✓ Slow the inflow slightly.
- ✓ Adjust patient position.
- ✓ Ask them to relax and breathe slowly.

Often, discomfort reduces within minutes.

**If There Is Sharp or Severe Pain**

This is not normal.

Immediately:

- ✓ Slow or stop inflow.
- ✓ Check tubing for kinks.
- ✓ Check clamp position.

Ask patient to change position slightly.
If pain continues:

- ✓ Stop the inflow.
- ✓ Contact your doctor.

Never ignore strong abdominal pain.

**Control the Speed of Inflow**

Do not allow fluid to rush in too fast.
Too rapid filling can cause:

- ✓ Sudden abdominal pressure
- ✓ Breathing discomfort
- ✓ Back pain

Keep it steady and controlled.
If necessary, slightly adjust clamp to slow flow.

**Expected Time for Inflow**

Usually inflow takes:
10 to 15 minutes
Time may vary depending on:

- ✓ Bag height
- ✓ Tubing length
- ✓ Patient position

If flow is very slow:

- ✓ Check for kinks.
- ✓ Ensure tube is fully broken.
- ✓ Raise solution bag slightly if required.

Do not shake or squeeze the bag forcefully.
Let gravity do the work.

**After Inflow Is Complete**

When all fresh solution has flowed in:

- ✓ Apply the blue clamp to seal the inflow tube.
- ✓ Close the white top mini cap securely.
- ✓ Ensure everything is properly sealed.
- ✓ Take a moment to check connections.

- ✓ Do not disconnect carelessly.

**Patient Position After Inflow**

Once filling is complete:

- ✓ Patient can move comfortably.
- ✓ Avoid sudden heavy movements.
- ✓ Encourage normal activity unless advised otherwise.

The fluid will now stay inside for the dwell period prescribed by the doctor.

**Common Mistakes during Inflow**

Avoid these:

- ✓ Forgetting to close caps before breaking tube
- ✓ Opening clamp too wide too quickly
- ✓ Ignoring patient discomfort
- ✓ Talking directly over open connections
- ✓ Allowing tubing to touch unclean surfaces
- ✓ Rushing to finish quickly

Calm, steady movements reduce risk.

**Emotional Reassurance During Inflow**

Some patients feel anxious during filling.
They may worry:
*"Is it too much fluid?""Why does it feel tight?"*
Speak calmly.
Explain gently:
*"This is the fresh solution. It will help clean your body."*
Reassurance reduces muscle tension — which reduces discomfort.

**Final Thoughts**

The inflow phase brings fresh cleansing fluid into the body.

It must be:
*Clean*
*Controlled*
*Calm*
When done properly, it should feel routine and safe.
Every exchange becomes easier with practice.
In the next chapter, we will cover the final step — completing the exchange safely and sealing everything properly to prevent contamination.
***Steady hands. Calm mind. Careful steps.***

# Chapter 10:
# Completing the Exchange Safely

**Finish Clean. Finish Calm. Finish Secure.**

You have drained the old fluid.

You have filled fresh solution.

Now comes the final and very important stage — completing the exchange properly.

Many caregivers relax once inflow is finished. But this last part is just as important as the beginning. A careless finish can undo careful preparation.

Think of it this way:

The exchange is only complete when everything is sealed, safe, and clean.

**Step 1: Applying the Blue Clamp**

Once the fresh solution has completely flowed in:

- ✓ Locate the inflow tubing.
- ✓ Apply the blue clamp firmly to seal the line.

Make sure:

- ✓ The clamp is fully closed.
- ✓ There is no fluid leakage.
- ✓ The tube is not twisted.

The blue clamp acts as a safety lock. It prevents any backflow and protects against contamination.

Do not leave the tubing unsecured.

Double-check visually.

A two-second check prevents future problems.

**Step 2: Sealing the Inflow Tube**

After applying the blue clamp:

- ✓ Ensure the white top cap is closed properly.
- ✓ Check that all connections are secure.
- ✓ Now carefully disconnect as per your training.

While disconnecting:

- ✓ Do not touch the open sterile ends.
- ✓ Keep movements slow and controlled.
- ✓ Avoid sudden jerks.

The goal is simple:
Seal everything without contamination.
If at any point you feel you accidentally touched a sterile area — stop and follow your infection control protocol.
Never ignore a suspected contamination.

**Step 3: Replacing the Mini Cap**

Now comes a very important protection step.
The catheter must always be sealed with a clean, sterile mini cap when not connected to dialysis tubing.
Steps:

- ✓ Remove the old mini cap (if required).
- ✓ Attach a new sterile mini cap.
- ✓ Tighten securely — but not forcefully.

The mini cap protects the catheter from:

- ✓ Air exposure
- ✓ Germs
- ✓ Accidental opening

Make sure:

- ✓ It is properly fitted.
- ✓ It does not feel loose.

The catheter is positioned comfortably.
Never reuse mini caps.
Always use a fresh sterile one.

**Step 4: Check the Weight of the Drained Fluid**

After every exchange, always check and record the weight of the drained fluid bag.

This step is very important. The weight tells you how much fluid has come out of the body. Since 1 gram equals approximately 1 millilitre, the weight of the drained fluid helps you understand whether excess fluid is being removed properly.

If the drained fluid weighs more than the amount of solution that went in, it means extra fluid has been removed from the body — this is usually good, especially if the patient has swelling or fluid overload.

If the drained fluid weighs less than expected, it may mean:

- ✓ Poor drainage
- ✓ Constipation affecting flow
- ✓ Catheter position issue
- ✓ Early sign of a blockage
- ✓ The body is retaining fluid

Regularly checking the drain weight helps:

- ✓ Monitor fluid balance
- ✓ Prevent fluid overload
- ✓ Avoid dehydration
- ✓ Detect problems early

Give accurate information to the PD team

Never skip this step. Write the weight clearly in your daily log. Patterns over several days are more important than one single reading.

If you notice a sudden big change (much less or much more than usual), inform your PD nurse or doctor.

This small habit can prevent big complications.

**Step 5: Disposal of Waste**

Once everything is sealed and secured, now focus on safe disposal.

**Drain Bag Disposal**

- ✓ Ensure drain bag is properly sealed.

- ✓ Check one final time for fluid clarity (if not already done).
- ✓ Fold and place it on the designated newspaper.
- ✓ Dispose according to medical guidance.
- ✓ Never pour drain fluid into random places unless instructed by your medical team.
- ✓ Follow your local medical waste disposal instructions.

**Used Supplies**

Discard:

- ✓ Syringes
- ✓ Used gauze
- ✓ Used gloves
- ✓ Used packaging
- ✓ Newspapers

Place them in a designated waste bag.

Seal and dispose properly.

Do not leave waste exposed.

**Post-Procedure Hygiene**

Even after the exchange is complete, hygiene continues.

**Remove Gloves Properly**

- ✓ Peel gloves from wrist downward.
- ✓ Avoid touching outer glove surface.
- ✓ Discard immediately.

**Wash Hands Again**

Yes — wash again.

After removing gloves:

- ✓ Perform proper handwashing.
- ✓ Dry thoroughly.
- ✓ Sanitize if required.

This protects both you and the patient.

**Clean the Area**

- ✓ Wipe the table again with sanitizer.
- ✓ Store unused supplies properly.
- ✓ Return equipment to its designated place.

A clean finish prepares you for the next exchange.

**Observe the Patient After Completion**

Do not immediately walk away.
Take a few minutes to check:

- ✓ Is the patient comfortable?
- ✓ Any unusual abdominal pain?
- ✓ Any dizziness?
- ✓ Any shortness of breath?

Mild fullness is normal.
Severe discomfort is not.
Encourage the patient to:

- ✓ Sit comfortably for a few minutes.
- ✓ Avoid sudden heavy lifting.
- ✓ Resume normal activities gradually.

**Emotional Closure After Exchange**

For many patients, exchanges can feel repetitive and tiring.
A small reassuring sentence helps:
*"Done for now. Everything went well."*
Routine reassurance builds confidence.

**Common Mistakes During Completion**

Avoid these common errors:

- ✓ Forgetting to apply blue clamp
- ✓ Not tightening mini cap properly
- ✓ Throwing away drain bag without checking fluid
- ✓ Leaving waste materials open
- ✓ Skipping final handwash

- ✓ Walking away without checking patient comfort

Completion deserves the same attention as preparation.

**Creating a Safe Habit**

When you complete every exchange with the same steps:

- ✓ *Clamp*
- ✓ *Seal*
- ✓ *Replace mini cap*
- ✓ *Weigh and Dispose*
- ✓ *Wash hands*
- ✓ *Check patient*

It becomes automatic.
*Routine reduces anxiety.*
*Routine increases safety.*

**Final Thoughts**

Finishing properly is a sign of responsible caregiving.
You are not just performing a task.
You are protecting a direct line into the abdomen — a space that must remain sterile.
Each safe completion builds confidence.
Each careful finish prevents infection.
You may not see the protection you provide — but it is working silently every day.

In the next chapter, we will move to daily exit site care and dressing protocol — another important area in preventing infection.
***Clean start. Clean process. Clean finish.***

# PART 5:
# ROUTINE CARE & DAILY MANAGEMENT

# Chapter 11:
# Exit Site Care & Dressing Protocol

**Protect the Entry. Protect the Life.**
The exit site is the small opening on the abdomen where the PD catheter comes out of the body.
It may look small.
But it is very important.
This tiny opening is a direct path into the abdomen. If germs enter here, infection can travel inside and cause serious complications like peritonitis.
That is why exit site care is not optional. t is daily protection.
Done properly, it keeps the catheter safe for years.

**Why Exit Site Care Matters**
The skin is our natural protection.
But where the catheter exits, that protection is slightly broken.
So we must:
- ✓ Keep it clean
- ✓ Keep it dry
- ✓ Keep it covered
- ✓ Check it daily

Even one careless day can increase infection risk.
Make exit site care a routine — like brushing teeth.

**Dressing Items (As Per SOP)**
Before starting, keep everything ready.
You should have:
- ✓ *Clean mask*
- ✓ *Sterile gloves*
- ✓ *Benzodine solution (Povidone-Iodine, if prescribed)*

- ✓ *Sterile gauze pieces*
- ✓ *Prescribed antibiotic ointment (T-Bact) (eg; Mupirocin) if doctor advised*
- ✓ *Transparent dressing tape*
- ✓ *Waste disposal bag*
- ✓ *Hand sanitizer*

Never start without arranging everything first.
Preparation prevents mistakes.

**Step 1: Prepare Yourself**

Before touching the exit site:

- ✓ *Wash hands properly using 6-step handwashing.*
- ✓ *Wear mask.*
- ✓ *Wear sterile gloves.*

Even if the site "looks fine," never skip these steps.
Remember — infection is invisible.

**Step 2: Remove Old Dressing Carefully**

- ✓ Gently remove the old gauze.
- ✓ Do not pull suddenly.
- ✓ Support the catheter while removing tape.
- ✓ Observe the old dressing.

Check if you see:

- ✓ Yellow discharge
- ✓ Blood spots
- ✓ Foul smell
- ✓ Wetness

If anything unusual is noticed, inform the doctor or PD nurse.
Dispose of old dressing safely.

**Step 3: Inspect the Exit Site**

Before cleaning, look carefully.
Healthy exit site should:

- ✓ Be dry
- ✓ Have no swelling
- ✓ Have no redness
- ✓ Have no pus
- ✓ Have no strong pain

Mild pink color can be normal in some patients.
But bright redness, warmth, or tenderness is not normal.
Ask the patient:
*"Is there pain when I touch here?"*
Pain is an early warning sign.

**Step 4: Cleaning with Benzodine**

Benzodine (Povidone-Iodine) is commonly used to clean the area, if prescribed.
How to clean:

- ✓ *Take sterile gauze.*
- ✓ *Pour small amount of Benzodine on it.*
- ✓ *Clean in circular motion.*
- ✓ *Always move from inside (near catheter) outward.*
- ✓ *Never go from outside inward.*
- ✓ *Use each gauze only once.*
- ✓ *Do not rub hard.*
- ✓ *Gentle cleaning is enough.*
- ✓ *Let the area air dry.*

Do not blow on it.
Do not fan it.
Drying is important before applying ointment.

**Step 5: Ointment Use (If Prescribed)**

Some patients are advised to apply antibiotic ointment *(T-Bact) (eg; Mupirocin)* daily.
If prescribed:

- ✓ Use clean sterile gauze.

- ✓ Apply a thin layer around the catheter site.
- ✓ Do not apply too much.
- ✓ More ointment does not mean better protection.
- ✓ Too much can make area moist — and moisture increases infection risk.
- ✓ If no ointment is prescribed, do not apply anything on your own.

No powders.
No home remedies.
No herbal pastes.
Only doctor-approved products.

**Step 6: Gauze Application**

Once the area is clean and dry:

- ✓ Place sterile gauze gently around the catheter.
- ✓ Ensure it covers the site completely.
- ✓ Do not press tightly.

The gauze should:

- ✓ Protect
- ✓ Absorb minor moisture
- ✓ Keep area clean

It should not suffocate the skin.

**Step 7: Transparent Tape Usage**

Now secure the gauze with transparent dressing tape.

Why transparent?

Because:

- ✓ It allows you to see the area.
- ✓ It holds dressing securely.
- ✓ It protects from outside contamination.

How to apply:

- ✓ Place tape smoothly.
- ✓ Avoid folds or air pockets.

- ✓ Do not stretch skin tightly.
- ✓ Make sure the catheter is supported and not hanging freely.
- ✓ Loose catheter movement causes irritation and infection.

It is advisable for patients to use catheter belts for support. Follow doctor's advice.

**Important Daily Rules**

- ✓ Keep exit site dry.
- ✓ Do not allow sweat to collect.
- ✓ Avoid tight clothing rubbing against site.
- ✓ Do not scratch.
- ✓ Do not pull catheter accidentally.
- ✓ Avoid bathing in tubs unless permitted.
- ✓ Avoid swimming unless doctor allows.

During shower:

- ✓ Cover site properly if advised.
- ✓ Dry immediately after.

Moisture is infection's friend.
Dryness is safety.

**Signs of Exit Site Infection**

Know these warning signs.
Contact doctor immediately if you see:

- ✓ Redness spreading around site
- ✓ Swelling
- ✓ Warm skin around catheter
- ✓ Yellow or green discharge
- ✓ Bad smell
- ✓ Pain on touch
- ✓ Fever

Never wait.
Early treatment prevents serious complications.

**Difference Between Exit Site Infection and Peritonitis**

Exit site infection:

- ✓ Local redness
- ✓ Discharge from skin area
- ✓ Pain at site

Peritonitis:

- ✓ Severe abdominal pain
- ✓ Cloudy drain fluid
- ✓ Fever
- ✓ Nausea

Both need medical attention.

**Common Caregiver Mistakes**

Avoid these:

- ✓ *Skipping daily inspection*
- ✓ *Cleaning without handwashing*
- ✓ *Using non-sterile cotton/ guaze*
- ✓ *Applying random creams*
- ✓ *Leaving site uncovered*
- ✓ *Reusing gauze*
- ✓ *Ignoring mild redness*

Small negligence becomes big infection.

**Emotional Care During Dressing**

Some patients feel sensitive about the catheter.
Be gentle.
Do not rush.
Speak calmly:
*"Just cleaning now."*
*"Almost done."*
*"Looks good today."*
Confidence reduces fear.

**Creating a Routine**

Best time for dressing:

- ✓ Same time daily
- ✓ In good lighting
- ✓ In a clean room

Consistency builds habit. Habit builds safety.

**Final Thoughts**

Exit site care may look simple.

But it is one of the most powerful infection prevention steps in PD care.

This small daily act protects:

The catheter

The abdomen

The patient's life

Do it with attention. Do it with discipline. Do it with care.

# Chapter 12:
# Daily Monitoring Checklist

**Small Daily Checks Prevent Big Problems**

Peritoneal dialysis does not end after the exchange is completed.

Daily monitoring is equally important.

Many complications do not happen suddenly.

They give small warning signs first.

If you watch carefully every day, you can detect problems early and prevent hospital visits.

This chapter will guide you on what to check daily, how to record it, and why it matters.

Make this your daily safety routine.

## 1. Weight Tracking

Weight is not just a number.

For PD patients, weight tells us about fluid balance.

**Why Weight Matters**

If weight suddenly increases:

→ It may mean fluid is building up inside the body.

If weight suddenly drops:

→ It may mean dehydration or poor nutrition.

**When to Check Weight**

- ✓ Every morning
- ✓ After passing urine
- ✓ Before eating breakfast
- ✓ Wearing similar light clothing
- ✓ Using the same weighing machine

Consistency is important.

**What to Record**

- ✓ Write down:
- ✓ Date
- ✓ Weight

- ✓ Any remarks (for example: swelling, poor appetite)

**When to Inform Doctor**

Call your PD nurse or doctor if:

- ✓ Weight increases more than 1 kg in one day
- ✓ Weight increases steadily for 2–3 days
- ✓ Weight drops suddenly with weakness or dizziness
- ✓ Weight changes often show fluid problems before swelling appears.

Never ignore sudden changes.

**2. Blood Pressure (BP) Monitoring**

Kidney patients often have BP problems.

PD can improve BP control, but monitoring is still necessary.

**When to Check BP**

Once daily (preferably morning)

Same time each day

Before dialysis exchange or as advised

If patient feels:

- ✓ Headache
- ✓ Dizziness
- ✓ Blurred vision
- ✓ Chest discomfort

Check BP immediately.

**What is Normal?**

The doctor will tell you the target range.

Usually:

- ✓ Very high BP needs attention.
- ✓ Very low BP can cause weakness or fainting.

**Record It**

- ✓ Write:
- ✓ Date
- ✓ Time

- ✓ BP reading
- ✓ Pulse rate (if machine shows)

Do not panic at one abnormal reading.
But repeated abnormal readings must be reported.

**3. Fluid Balance Chart**

Fluid balance means:
How much fluid goes IN Versus How much fluid comes OUT. This is very important in PD.

**Fluid Intake Includes:**

- ✓ Drinking water
- ✓ Tea, coffee
- ✓ Milk
- ✓ Soup
- ✓ Juice
- ✓ Ice cream
- ✓ Watery fruits (like watermelon)

Everything liquid counts.

**Fluid Output Includes:**

Urine
PD drain output

**Why It Matters**

If intake is too much: → Swelling, breathlessness, high BP.
If intake is too little: → Dehydration, low BP, cramps.
Maintain the balance advised by the doctor.

**4. Intake–Output Record**

Keep a notebook dedicated only for PD monitoring.
Create simple columns:
Date | Fluid Intake | Urine Output | PD Drain Volume | Remarks

**Example:**

Intake: 1200 ml
Urine: 400 ml

PD drain: 2000 ml
Doctor uses these numbers to adjust PD strength.
Never guess numbers.
Use a measuring jar for accuracy.
Even small mistakes can change treatment decisions.

**5. Swelling Check (Edema Monitoring)**
Swelling is a common sign of fluid overload.
Check daily for:

- ✓ Swollen feet
- ✓ Swollen ankles
- ✓ Puffy face
- ✓ Tight rings on fingers
- ✓ Tight shoes
- ✓ Abdominal bloating

Press gently over ankle bone.
If dent remains for a few seconds:→ It may be fluid retention.
Also observe:

- ✓ Sudden breathlessness
- ✓ Difficulty lying flat

These are serious signs. Inform doctor immediately.

**6. Appetite Observation**
Appetite tells a lot about overall health.
Healthy PD patients should maintain reasonable appetite.
Watch for:

- ✓ Refusing food
- ✓ Feeling full quickly
- ✓ Nausea
- ✓ Vomiting
- ✓ Weight loss
- ✓ Weakness

Poor appetite may mean:

- ✓ Infection
- ✓ Peritonitis
- ✓ Depression
- ✓ Uremia
- ✓ Electrolyte imbalance

Never ignore poor appetite for many days.
Nutrition is strength.
Strength supports recovery.

**Daily Monitoring Summary Checklist**

Every Day, Ask:

✓ *Did I check weight?*
✓ *Did I check BP?*
✓ *Did I record fluid intake?*
✓ *Did I record output?*
✓ *Did I check swelling?*
✓ *Did I observe appetite?*
✓ *Did I observe mood and energy level?*

This takes only 10–15 minutes.
But it can prevent emergencies.

**When to Call Doctor Immediately**

Call without delay if you notice:

- ✓ Sudden weight gain
- ✓ Severe swelling
- ✓ Breathlessness
- ✓ Very high BP
- ✓ Very low BP with fainting
- ✓ No urine output suddenly
- ✓ Cloudy drain fluid
- ✓ Fever
- ✓ Severe abdominal pain
- ✓ Continuous vomiting

Do not wait for the next appointment.

Early reporting saves life.

**Emotional Monitoring Is Also Important**

PD patients sometimes feel:

- ✓ Tired
- ✓ Irritated
- ✓ Sad
- ✓ Hopeless

Caregiver should gently observe mood changes. Encourage conversation. Sometimes emotional support is as important as medical care.

**Creating a Monitoring Routine**

Keep:

- ✓ One dedicated notebook
- ✓ One pen attached to it
- ✓ Keep it near PD station
- ✓ Never rely on memory.
- ✓ Write everything.
- ✓ Doctors trust written records.

Written records guide safe treatment.

**Final Words**

Daily monitoring may feel repetitive. But repetition creates safety.

These small daily checks are not "extra work." They are protection.

Protection of:

- ✓ The catheter
- ✓ The kidneys
- ✓ The heart
- ✓ The patient's life

A careful caregiver is a silent lifesaver.

# Chapter 13:
# Nutrition & Fluid Discipline

Food Is Not Just Taste — It Is Treatment

For a patient on Peritoneal Dialysis (PD), food is not just about hunger.

Food becomes part of treatment.

What the patient eats and drinks directly affects:

- ✓ Blood pressure
- ✓ Swelling
- ✓ Energy levels
- ✓ Blood sugar
- ✓ Infection risk
- ✓ Overall survival

Many caregivers focus only on dialysis exchange.

But daily food discipline is equally important.

This chapter will help you understand what to give, what to limit, and why it matters.

## 1. Salt Restriction

Less Salt = Less Swelling

Salt makes the body hold water.

When kidneys are weak, they cannot remove extra salt properly.

Extra salt leads to:

- ✓ *Swelling in legs*
- ✓ *Puffy face*
- ✓ *High blood pressure*
- ✓ *Breathlessness*
- ✓ *Increased fluid overload*

**Where Salt Hides**

Salt is not only in table salt.

It is also hidden in:

- ✓ Pickles

- ✓ Papad
- ✓ Chips
- ✓ Bakery items
- ✓ Namkeen snacks
- ✓ Processed foods
- ✓ Sauces
- ✓ Ready-made soups
- ✓ Even biscuits may contain salt.

**Practical Tips**

Do not keep salt shaker on the table.
Cook with less salt.
Avoid packaged snacks.
Use jeera, dhania for taste.
Taste food before adding extra salt.
Family members should also adjust.
If one person eats low salt and others eat normally, it becomes difficult emotionally.
Support the patient by eating similar food.

**2. Protein Importance**

Protein Is Healing Food
Many people think kidney patients should avoid protein.
This is partly true for some stages.
But PD patients actually lose protein through dialysis fluid daily.
So protein becomes very important.
Without enough protein, patient may develop:

- ✓ Weakness
- ✓ Poor immunity
- ✓ Slow wound healing
- ✓ Hair fall
- ✓ Low albumin levels

**Good Protein Sources**

(As per doctor's advice)

- ✓ Egg whites
- ✓ Fish
- ✓ Chicken
- ✓ Paneer
- ✓ Milk (in controlled quantity)
- ✓ Dal (as permitted)
- ✓ Sprouts (if potassium allows)

**Signs of Low Protein**

- ✓ Weakness
- ✓ Swelling due to low albumin
- ✓ Muscle loss
- ✓ Frequent infections

Do not reduce protein unnecessarily.
Always follow dietician guidance.
Protein builds strength. Strength fights infection.

**3. Potassium Caution**

Too Much Potassium Can Be Dangerous. Potassium affects the heart.
High potassium can cause:

- ✓ Muscle weakness
- ✓ Irregular heartbeat
- ✓ Even cardiac arrest

PD removes potassium, but levels must still be monitored.

**High Potassium Foods (Limit if advised)**

- ✓ Banana
- ✓ Orange
- ✓ Coconut water
- ✓ Potato
- ✓ Tomato
- ✓ Spinach
- ✓ Dry fruits
- ✓ Avocado

**Lower Potassium Options**

- ✓ Apple
- ✓ Papaya (small portions)
- ✓ Cabbage
- ✓ Bottle gourd
- ✓ Ridge gourd

**Cooking Tip**

For vegetables like potato:

Cut into small pieces. Soak in water for few hours. Boil and discard water. Then cook.

This reduces potassium content.

Never follow random internet diet advice.

Always check blood reports and follow doctor instructions.

## 4. Fluid Restrictions

Too Much Fluid Is Dangerous

PD removes fluid, but there is still a limit to how much a patient should drink.

Excess fluid leads to:

- ✓ Swelling
- ✓ Breathlessness
- ✓ High BP
- ✓ Heart strain

**What Counts as Fluid?**

Everything liquid counts:

- ✓ Water
- ✓ Tea
- ✓ Coffee
- ✓ Milk
- ✓ Soup
- ✓ Ice cream
- ✓ Juice
- ✓ Buttermilk
- ✓ Even watery fruits

- ✓ Even ice cubes count.

**How to Control Thirst**

Patients often feel thirsty.

Try:

- ✓ Small sips instead of large glasses
- ✓ Rinse mouth without swallowing
- ✓ Chew sugar-free gum (if allowed)
- ✓ Use small cup instead of large glass
- ✓ Avoid salty foods (they increase thirst)

Measure daily intake.

Do not guess.

Fluid discipline prevents hospital admission.

**5. Diabetes Considerations**

PD Fluid Contains Sugar

PD solution contains glucose (sugar).

This means:

- ✓ Blood sugar can rise.
- ✓ Diabetic patients need closer monitoring.

**Important Points**

- ✓ Check blood sugar regularly.
- ✓ Inform doctor if sugar readings increase.
- ✓ Insulin dose may need adjustment.
- ✓ Do not skip diabetes medication.

**Diet Tips for Diabetic PD Patients**

- ✓ Avoid sweets.
- ✓ Avoid sugary drinks.
- ✓ Limit white rice quantity.
- ✓ Choose high-fiber foods.
- ✓ Eat small frequent meals.

PD itself may increase appetite because toxins are removed. But overeating causes weight gain and sugar problems. Balance is important.

**Signs That Diet Needs Review**

Call doctor or dietician if:

- ✓ Sudden weight gain
- ✓ Persistent swelling
- ✓ Poor appetite
- ✓ High potassium in blood test
- ✓ Low albumin levels
- ✓ Poor blood sugar control

Do not make sudden diet changes without guidance.

**Emotional Side of Food Discipline**

Food is emotional. Patient may feel:

- ✓ Frustrated
- ✓ Restricted
- ✓ Angry
- ✓ Sad

Especially when others eat freely.

As caregiver:

- ✓ Do not scold.
- ✓ Do not shame.
- ✓ Do not compare.

Instead say:

*"This food is helping your body stay strong."*

Encourage small treats occasionally — as per doctor's permission.

Balance medical discipline with emotional understanding.

**Sample Daily Balanced Approach (General Idea)**

Morning:

- ✓ Egg white / controlled breakfast
- ✓ Measured tea

Lunch:

- ✓ Controlled rice or chapati
- ✓ One protein source

- ✓ Low-salt vegetables

Evening:

- ✓ Light snack (non-salty)

Dinner:

- ✓ Light meal
- ✓ Avoid heavy late-night eating

This is only a general example.
Follow personalized diet plan from doctor.

**Common Caregiver Mistakes**

Avoid:

- ✓ Forcing patient to eat very little
- ✓ Over-restricting protein
- ✓ Ignoring salt in packaged food
- ✓ Giving coconut water without checking potassium
- ✓ Allowing unlimited fluids on "good days"
- ✓ Ignoring rising blood sugar

Consistency is more important than strictness.

**Final Thoughts**

Food can heal.
Food can harm.
For a PD patient, diet is not punishment. It is protection.

- ✓ When salt is controlled,
- ✓ When protein is adequate,
- ✓ When potassium is monitored,
- ✓ When fluids are disciplined,
- ✓ When diabetes is managed,

The patient remains stable, energetic, and safer.
Caregiver's kitchen becomes part of the dialysis machine.

# PART 6:
# PRECAUTIONS & EMERGENCIES

# Chapter 14:
# Do's & Don'ts for PD Caregivers

Discipline Today Prevents Emergency Tomorrow
Peritoneal Dialysis at home is safe.
But it is safe only when discipline is maintained.
PD does not forgive carelessness.
A small mistake at the connection point can cause infection. A missed warning sign can lead to hospitalization.
This chapter is not to frighten you. It is to protect you.
Keep these Do's and Don'ts visible near your PD station.
They are your daily safety reminders.

**DO'S FOR PD CAREGIVERS**

**1. Maintain Sterile Discipline**

Sterile discipline means:

- ✓ Clean hands every time.
- ✓ Mask before exchange.
- ✓ Gloves during dressing and exchange.
- ✓ Clean surface before placing items.
- ✓ Even if you are in a hurry — never skip handwashing.
- ✓ Even if you "just washed" — wash again before touching connections.

Infection does not announce itself. It enters quietly. Your discipline blocks its entry.

**2. Always Check the PD Solution**

Before every exchange, check:

- ✓ Correct strength (as prescribed)
- ✓ Correct volume
- ✓ Expiry date

- ✓ No leaks
- ✓ No cloudiness
- ✓ No damage to bag
- ✓ No broken seals
- ✓ Hold the bag against light.
- ✓ The solution should be clear.
- ✓ Never assume it is fine.
- ✓ Always check.

One careless exchange can introduce infection or wrong fluid balance.

**3. Keep Emergency Numbers Ready**

Do not search for numbers during panic.

Keep written clearly near PD station:

- ✓ PD doctor number
- ✓ PD nurse number
- ✓ Hospital emergency number
- ✓ Ambulance number
- ✓ Nearest emergency facility

Save them in mobile phones also. But also keep written copy. In emergency, phones may not be accessible immediately. Preparation reduces fear.

**4. Record Abnormalities Immediately**

If you notice:

- ✓ Cloudy drain fluid
- ✓ Blood in drain fluid
- ✓ Fever
- ✓ Abdominal pain
- ✓ Reduced drain amount
- ✓ Weight gain
- ✓ Swelling
- ✓ High BP
- ✓ Poor appetite

Write it down. Note time and date.

When you speak to doctor, clear information helps faster decisions.

Do not depend on memory. Documentation saves time. Time saves life.

**5. Observe the Patient Daily**

Look at:

- ✓ Energy level
- ✓ Mood
- ✓ Appetite
- ✓ Swelling
- ✓ Exit site condition
- ✓ Drain color
- ✓ Sometimes patients hide discomfort.
- ✓ Observe quietly.
- ✓ Small early signs are easier to treat.

**6. Maintain Routine**

PD works best when routine is followed.

- ✓ Same exchange timing daily
- ✓ Same cleaning discipline
- ✓ Same monitoring time

Irregular routine increases mistakes.

Routine creates safety.

**DON'TS FOR PD CAREGIVERS**

**1. Never Touch Connection Points**

This is extremely important.

Connection points must remain sterile.

Never:

- ✓ Touch them with bare hands.
- ✓ Allow them to touch table.
- ✓ Allow them to touch clothes.
- ✓ Allow them to hang loosely.

If accidental touch happens: Stop!

Do not continue casually.
Follow emergency protocol or inform PD nurse.
One touch can introduce bacteria.

**2. Never Reuse Disposable Items**

Do not reuse:

- ✓ Gloves
- ✓ Gauze
- ✓ Minicaps
- ✓ Masks
- ✓ Tubing
- ✓ Any disposable sterile item

Even if it "looks clean." Disposable means single use.
Reusing increases infection risk.
Do not try to save money in this area. Hospital admission costs much more.

**3. Never Ignore Cloudy Drain Fluid**

Cloudy fluid is not normal. It is often the first sign of peritonitis.
If drain fluid looks:

- ✓ Milky
- ✓ Hazy
- ✓ Thick
- ✓ With floating particles

Call doctor immediately. Do not wait for fever. Do not wait for pain.
Early treatment can prevent serious complications.

**4. Never Delay Doctor Communication**

Many caregivers wait.
They think:
*"Let us see tomorrow." "It may improve." "Maybe it is small issue."*
Do not delay.

In PD care:
Early reporting is wisdom. Late reporting is risk. Doctors prefer early calls rather than late emergencies.

**5. Never Perform Exchange in Unclean Area**
Do not:

- ✓ Sit near open windows with dust
- ✓ Use fan blowing directly
- ✓ Allow pets near area
- ✓ Allow children to touch items
- ✓ Do exchange in crowded room

Choose quiet, clean, well-lit space. PD needs controlled environment.

**6. Never Skip Exit Site Care**
Even if patient feels tired. Even if you are busy.
Daily dressing protects catheter. Skipping increases infection risk. No compromise.

**7. Never Guess Medication Doses**
Do not change:

- ✓ Antibiotics
- ✓ Heparin
- ✓ BP tablets
- ✓ Insulin
- ✓ PD fluid strength

Without doctor instruction. If unsure — ask. Do not experiment.

**Red Flag Situations (Immediate Medical Attention Needed)**
Call doctor urgently if:

- ✓ Severe abdominal pain
- ✓ Cloudy drain fluid

- ✓ Fever
- ✓ Vomiting
- ✓ No drain outflow
- ✓ Sudden swelling with breathlessness
- ✓ Very high BP
- ✓ Very low BP with fainting

Do not wait for routine appointment.

**Emotional Do's & Don'ts**

PD patients may feel:

- ✓ Dependent
- ✓ Embarrassed
- ✓ Frustrated
- ✓ Fearful

Do:

- ✓ Speak calmly
- ✓ Encourage
- ✓ Appreciate their cooperation

Don't:

- ✓ Blame them for complications
- ✓ Show anger during mistakes
- ✓ Make them feel like a burden

Healing also needs emotional strength.

**A Simple Golden Rule**

If you are ever unsure about anything: Pause!
Do not continue blindly. Call and clarify.
Better to ask twice than regret once.

**Final Words**

Being a PD caregiver is a responsibility. But it is also an act of love.

- ✓ Your careful hands protect the patient every day.
- ✓ Your discipline prevents infection.

- ✓ Your observation prevents emergencies.
- ✓ Your calm voice reduces fear.

Follow these Do's. Avoid these Don'ts.

And PD at home can remain safe, stable, and successful.

# Chapter 15: Complications & What To Do

**Stay Calm. Act Early. Save Time.**

Peritoneal Dialysis is safe when done properly. But like any medical treatment, problems can sometimes happen.

Do not panic when you hear the word "complication."

Most problems can be treated successfully — if detected early.

Your job as a caregiver is not to treat the complication yourself.

Your job is to:

- ✓ Recognize early signs
- ✓ Stay calm
- ✓ Inform the doctor quickly
- ✓ Follow instructions properly

This chapter explains common complications in simple language and what you should do immediately.

## 1. Peritonitis

The Most Important Emergency to Recognize

Peritonitis means infection inside the abdomen. It is the most serious complication in PD.

**Early Signs of Peritonitis**

- ✓ *Cloudy drain fluid (milky appearance)*
- ✓ *Abdominal pain*
- ✓ *Fever*
- ✓ *Nausea or vomiting*
- ✓ *Weakness*
- ✓ *Sometimes chills*

Very often, cloudy fluid appears before fever.

Never ignore cloudy fluid.

**What To Do Immediately**

- ✓ Stop and observe the drained fluid carefully.
- ✓ Do not throw it away immediately if doctor needs to see sample.
- ✓ Call the PD doctor or nurse immediately.
- ✓ Follow instructions — they may ask you to come to hospital.

Do not:

- ✓ Wait for pain to increase.
- ✓ Take home antibiotics without prescription.
- ✓ Ignore mild symptoms.
- ✓ Early treatment usually saves the catheter.

Delay can lead to serious infection and hospitalization.

**2. Hernia**

When Pressure Pushes Outward

Hernia happens when internal pressure causes a bulge in the abdomen or groin area.

PD fluid inside the abdomen increases pressure.

**Signs of Hernia**

- ✓ Swelling or bulge near belly button
- ✓ Groin swelling
- ✓ Pain when standing
- ✓ Swelling increases when coughing
- ✓ Sometimes it is painless at first.

**What To Do**

- ✓ Inform the doctor.
- ✓ Do not ignore swelling.
- ✓ Doctor may adjust fluid volume.
- ✓ In some cases, surgery may be required.

Do not:

- ✓ Lift heavy objects.
- ✓ Strain during constipation.
- ✓ Ignore early signs.

Prevent constipation with proper diet and doctor-approved medicines.

### 3. Leakage Around Exit Site

Fluid Coming Out Where It Should Not Sometimes PD fluid may leak around the catheter site.

**Signs**

- ✓ Wet dressing repeatedly
- ✓ Clear fluid around exit site
- ✓ Feeling of wetness after filling

**What To Do**

- ✓ Inform doctor immediately.
- ✓ Do not continue normal exchange without advice.
- ✓ Doctor may reduce fill volume temporarily.
- ✓ Extra rest may be advised.

Do not:

- ✓ Tighten dressing forcefully.
- ✓ Ignore continuous wetness.

Early correction prevents infection.

### 4. Blocked Catheter

When Fluid Does Not Flow Properly Sometimes drain fluid does not come out properly. Or inflow becomes very slow.

**Signs**

- ✓ Very slow draining
- ✓ No drain output
- ✓ Abdominal fullness
- ✓ Pain during inflow

**Common Reasons**

- ✓ Constipation
- ✓ Catheter tip position change
- ✓ Fibrin blocking tube
- ✓ Kink in tubing

**What To Do**

First:

- ✓ Check tubing for kinks.
- ✓ Ask patient to change position.
- ✓ Ask patient to cough gently.
- ✓ Ask patient to sit up or lie on side.

If still not draining:

- ✓ Call the doctor.
- ✓ Often constipation is the cause.
- ✓ Managing bowel movement daily is very important in PD patients.

Never ignore constipation.

**5. Fluid Overload**

Too Much Fluid in the Body

This happens when excess fluid builds up.

**Signs of Fluid Overload**

- ✓ Swelling in feet and face
- ✓ Sudden weight gain
- ✓ Breathlessness
- ✓ Tight clothes
- ✓ Reduced urine output
- ✓ High BP

**What To Do**

- ✓ Check weight immediately.
- ✓ Review fluid intake.
- ✓ Inform doctor.
- ✓ Doctor may increase PD strength temporarily.

Do not:

- ✓ Increase PD strength on your own.
- ✓ Ignore breathlessness.

Fluid overload can strain the heart.

**6. Dehydration**

Too Little Fluid in the Body

Sometimes too much fluid is removed.

**Signs of Dehydration**

- ✓ Dizziness
- ✓ Dry mouth
- ✓ Weakness
- ✓ Low BP
- ✓ Muscle cramps
- ✓ Rapid heartbeat

**What To Do**

- ✓ Check BP.
- ✓ Inform doctor.
- ✓ Doctor may reduce PD strength.
- ✓ Increase fluid intake only if advised.

Do not:

- ✓ Continue high-strength PD fluid blindly.
- ✓ Ignore repeated dizziness.

Balance is key.

- ✓ Too much fluid is dangerous.
- ✓ Too little fluid is also dangerous.

**7. Hypotension (Low Blood Pressure)**

Low BP can make patient feel faint or weak.

**Symptoms**

- ✓ Dizziness
- ✓ Blurred vision
- ✓ Sweating
- ✓ Fainting feeling
- ✓ Extreme weakness

**Causes in PD**

- ✓ Dehydration
- ✓ Excess fluid removal
- ✓ Infection

Blood pressure medication adjustment needed

**What To Do**

- ✓ Make patient lie down.

- ✓ Raise legs slightly.
- ✓ Check BP.
- ✓ Inform doctor if BP is very low or symptoms persist.

Do not:

- ✓ Force patient to stand quickly.
- ✓ Ignore repeated episodes.

**When To Go To Hospital Immediately**

Do not delay hospital visit if:

- ✓ *Severe abdominal pain*
- ✓ *High fever*
- ✓ *Continuous vomiting*
- ✓ *Severe breathlessness*
- ✓ *No urine output suddenly*
- ✓ *Fainting*
- ✓ *Severe swelling*
- ✓ *Chest pain*

Trust your instinct. If something feels seriously wrong, seek help.

**Emotional Side of Complications**

Complications create fear.

Patient may feel:

*"Why is this happening to me?" "Will I need to stop PD?" "Will I need surgery?"*

As caregiver:

- ✓ Stay calm.
- ✓ Your calmness reassures the patient.

Most complications are treatable. PD can continue safely after proper treatment.

**The Golden Rule**

In PD care:

- ✓ Early detection

- ✓ Early reporting
- ✓ Early treatment

These three prevent disaster. Never hide problems. Never delay communication.

**Final Thoughts**

Complications are not failure. They are signals. Signals that something needs adjustment. Your role is not to solve everything alone. Your role is to notice early and act responsibly.

With careful monitoring, timely communication, and calm handling, most complications can be managed successfully.

# PART 7:
# EMOTIONAL & LONG-TERM SUPPORT

# Chapter 16:
# Supporting the Patient Emotionally

**Healing the Mind While Caring for the Body**

Peritoneal Dialysis treats the body. But kidney failure affects the mind. Many patients look normal from outside. But inside, they may be carrying fear, frustration, and silent sadness. As a caregiver, you are not just managing exchanges.

You are supporting a human being going through a life change.

This chapter will help you understand the emotional side of PD — and how to support both the patient and yourself.

## 1. Anxiety Management

Fear Is Common — and Normal. Most PD patients worry about:

- ✓ Infection
- ✓ Doing something wrong
- ✓ Becoming dependent
- ✓ Financial burden
- ✓ Future health
- ✓ Hospital admissions

Some do not speak openly about their fears.

They may become quiet or irritable instead.

**Signs of Anxiety**

- ✓ Restlessness
- ✓ Poor sleep
- ✓ Irritation
- ✓ Repeated questions
- ✓ Fear before exchanges
- ✓ Negative thinking

**How You Can Help**

Speak calmly during procedures. A calm voice reduces fear. Explain each step gently. *"Now we are connecting." "Drain is starting." "Everything looks clear."*

Encourage questions. Do not dismiss their worries. Avoid medical jargon. Use simple explanations. Keep routine stable. Routine reduces uncertainty. Remind them of progress. *"You've been doing well." "Your reports improved."*

Sometimes just listening quietly helps more than advice.

**2. Fatigue Support**

Kidney Disease Is Tiring Even with PD, many patients feel tired.

Fatigue may be due to:

- ✓ Anemia
- ✓ Poor sleep
- ✓ Emotional stress
- ✓ Nutritional imbalance
- ✓ Chronic illness itself

**Signs of Fatigue**

- ✓ Sleeping more than usual
- ✓ Lack of interest
- ✓ Irritability
- ✓ Slow movements
- ✓ Low motivation

**What You Can Do**

Encourage short walks (if doctor permits). Plan activities during their best energy time. Allow rest without guilt. Ensure proper nutrition. Check blood tests regularly (as advised).

Do not say: *"You are always tired." "Others are worse than you."*

Instead say: *"Let's take it slowly." "Rest for some time." "We'll manage together."*
Small encouragement builds strength.

### 3. Encouragement & Positive Reinforcement

Words Can Heal. Chronic illness sometimes affects self-esteem.

The patient may feel:

- ✓ Less independent
- ✓ A burden to family
- ✓ Different from others

As caregiver, your words matter deeply.

**Simple Encouragement Examples**

*"You are managing very well."*
*"Your discipline is helping your health."*
*"We are proud of your strength."*
*"This is just one part of life, not the whole of life."*

Celebrate small victories:

- ✓ Stable blood reports
- ✓ Clear drain fluid
- ✓ Weight control
- ✓ Good BP readings

A small celebration can be:

- ✓ A favorite permitted meal
- ✓ Watching a movie together
- ✓ Calling a friend

Hope is powerful medicine.

### 4. Maintaining Social Connection

PD patients sometimes isolate themselves. They may feel embarrassed about the catheter.

Encourage:

- ✓ Safe social visits
- ✓ Phone calls
- ✓ Light outings (if medically stable)

- ✓ Hobbies

Life should not become only about dialysis. Dialysis is part of life — not the whole life.

**5. Avoiding Caregiver Burnout**

You Matter Too

Caregivers often forget themselves. They focus fully on the patient.

But caregiving can cause:

- ✓ *Physical exhaustion*
- ✓ *Emotional stress*
- ✓ *Irritation*
- ✓ *Sleep problems*
- ✓ *Feeling overwhelmed*

If caregiver collapses, patient care suffers.

**Signs of Caregiver Burnout**

- ✓ Constant tiredness
- ✓ Short temper
- ✓ Feeling unappreciated
- ✓ Crying easily
- ✓ Losing interest in personal activities

**How To Protect Yourself**

Take small breaks.

- ✓ Share responsibility when possible.
- ✓ Ask family members for support.
- ✓ Speak openly about your stress.
- ✓ Maintain your own health checkups.
- ✓ Sleep properly.

You are not selfish for resting. You are responsible.

**6. Communication Between Patient & Caregiver**

Healthy communication reduces tension.

Avoid:

- ✓ Blaming
- ✓ Shouting during procedures

- ✓ Bringing up old mistakes
- ✓ Comparing with other patients

Instead:

- ✓ Discuss concerns calmly.
- ✓ Plan together.
- ✓ Make decisions jointly.

PD is teamwork. Not authority.

**7. Handling Difficult Days**

Some days will be harder.

There may be:

- ✓ Cloudy fluid
- ✓ Poor reports
- ✓ Mood swings
- ✓ Hospital visits

On those days:

Focus only on one step at a time. Do not think too far ahead.

Say: *"We will handle today."*

One day at a time reduces mental pressure.

**8. Encouraging Independence**

If patient is capable, allow them to:

- ✓ Participate in exchange
- ✓ Maintain their own records
- ✓ Prepare dressing items
- ✓ Monitor BP

Involvement builds confidence. Overprotection can reduce morale.

Support — but do not control.

**9. When Professional Help Is Needed**

If patient shows:

- ✓ Continuous sadness
- ✓ Loss of interest in everything

- ✓ Refusal to eat
- ✓ Talking about hopelessness
- ✓ Severe anxiety
- ✓ Sleep problems for weeks

Consult a doctor.

Mental health is also health. There is no shame in seeking counseling.

**Final Thoughts**

Peritoneal Dialysis is not just a medical journey. It is an emotional journey for both patient and caregiver.

- ✓ There will be fear.
- ✓ There will be fatigue.
- ✓ There will be moments of frustration.

But there can also be strength, bonding, discipline, and resilience.

Support with patience. Speak with kindness. Rest when needed. Encourage daily.

Healing is not only about clear fluid.

It is about a peaceful mind and hopeful heart.

# Chapter 17:
# Long-Term Lifestyle with PD

**Living Fully — Not Just Surviving**

When a patient first starts Peritoneal Dialysis, everything feels new and overwhelming.

Over time, PD becomes part of daily routine.

Life does not stop because of dialysis. It simply needs planning.

With proper organization and confidence, a patient on PD can:

- ✓ Travel
- ✓ Attend family functions
- ✓ Celebrate festivals
- ✓ Continue work (if medically stable)
- ✓ Live with dignity

This chapter will guide you on managing long-term living with PD safely and confidently.

**1. Travel Planning**

Yes, Travel Is Possible — With Preparation

Many families believe that PD means staying home forever. That is not true.

PD is actually more flexible than hospital dialysis — but it requires planning.

**Before Planning Travel**

First ask:

- ✓ Is the patient medically stable?
- ✓ Has there been any recent infection?
- ✓ Are blood reports stable?
- ✓ Has the doctor approved travel?

Never plan travel without doctor's approval.

**Planning Short Trips (1–3 Days)**

For short travel:

- ✓ Carry extra PD bags (more than required)
- ✓ Carry dressing supplies
- ✓ Carry masks, gloves, minicap
- ✓ Carry sanitizer
- ✓ Carry emergency contact numbers
- ✓ Carry latest medical reports
- ✓ Always carry extra supplies.

Delays can happen. Never pack "exact quantity."

**Planning Longer Travel**

For longer trips:

- ✓ Inform PD unit in advance.
- ✓ Arrange delivery of PD supplies at destination if possible.
- ✓ Identify nearest hospital with dialysis facility.
- ✓ Keep doctor's letter explaining PD treatment.
- ✓ Carry prescription copy.

If traveling by air:

- ✓ Inform airline in advance.
- ✓ Carry medical certificate.
- ✓ Keep essential supplies in hand luggage.

Do not put critical supplies in check-in baggage.

**During Travel**

- ✓ Maintain hand hygiene strictly.
- ✓ Choose clean private area for exchange.
- ✓ Avoid crowded, dusty places.
- ✓ Keep pets away in holiday homes.
- ✓ Maintain timing discipline.
- ✓ Do not skip exchanges because of sightseeing.

*Health first.*

**2. Storage Management**

Organized Storage Prevents Mistakes PD supplies require proper storage.

Poor storage can damage solutions and increase infection risk.

**Where To Store PD Supplies**

Choose a:

- ✓ Clean room
- ✓ Dry space
- ✓ Cool area (room temperature)
- ✓ Away from direct sunlight
- ✓ Away from moisture

Do not store near:

- ✓ Bathroom
- ✓ Kitchen stove
- ✓ Damp walls
- ✓ Open windows

Keep boxes off the floor if possible. Use shelves or wooden pallets.

**Organizing Supplies**

Keep supplies arranged by:

- ✓ Expiry date (use older first)
- ✓ Fluid strength
- ✓ Daily requirement
- ✓ Label shelves if needed.

Keep:

- ✓ Dressing items separate
- ✓ Exchange items separate
- ✓ Emergency items easily accessible

Good storage reduces confusion during exchange.

**Monthly Stock Check**

- ✓ Once every month:
- ✓ Count remaining PD bags.
- ✓ Check expiry dates.
- ✓ Check for damaged packaging.
- ✓ Inform supplier in advance for next delivery.
- ✓ Never wait until the last minute.
- ✓ Always maintain buffer stock.

### 3. Hospital Coordination

Stay Connected With Your PD Team. Even if everything is stable, regular follow-up is important. PD is home-based — but medical supervision continues.

**Regular Follow-Ups**

Follow doctor's schedule for:

- ✓ Blood tests
- ✓ PET test (if required)
- ✓ Hemoglobin monitoring
- ✓ Albumin levels
- ✓ Electrolyte levels

Never skip appointments because patient feels fine. Regular review prevents future complications.

**Informing Hospital About Changes**

Always inform doctor if:

- ✓ Repeated BP changes
- ✓ Frequent swelling
- ✓ Weight fluctuations
- ✓ Poor appetite
- ✓ Emotional changes
- ✓ Exit site redness
- ✓ Even small changes matter.

Your doctor adjusts treatment based on these reports.

**Emergency Coordination**

Know:

- ✓ Nearest emergency hospital
- ✓ Backup PD nurse contact
- ✓ What to do if doctor unavailable

Preparation reduces fear.

**4. Maintaining Dignity**

The Patient Is More Than a Diagnosis. Chronic illness can affect dignity.

The patient may feel:

- ✓ Dependent
- ✓ Weak
- ✓ Different
- ✓ Embarrassed about catheter

As caregiver, protect their dignity.

**Simple Ways To Maintain Dignity**

- ✓ Knock before entering their room.
- ✓ Allow privacy during dressing.
- ✓ Involve them in decisions.
- ✓ Speak respectfully.
- ✓ Do not discuss their illness publicly without consent.

Even during procedures:

- ✓ Explain before touching.
- ✓ Respect builds confidence.

**5. Encouraging Independence**

Support Without Overpowering

If the patient is capable:

- ✓ Allow them to wash hands themselves.
- ✓ Let them record weight.
- ✓ Let them check BP.
- ✓ Let them assist during exchange.

Independence builds self-respect. Overprotection can create helplessness.

Support gently — do not control completely.

**6. Continuing Work & Social Life**

If medically stable, many PD patients can:

- ✓ Work part-time
- ✓ Manage business

- ✓ Attend social gatherings
- ✓ Travel locally
- ✓ Continue hobbies

Encourage normal activities within safety limits. Life should not revolve only around dialysis.

**7. Building Long-Term Confidence**

In the beginning, PD feels complicated. After a few months, it becomes routine.

Confidence grows when:

- ✓ Infection is prevented
- ✓ Monitoring is consistent
- ✓ Communication with doctor is clear
- ✓ Routine is disciplined

Remind the patient: *"You have managed this well."* Confidence reduces anxiety.

**8. Planning for the Future**

Discuss future openly:

- ✓ Transplant options (if applicable)
- ✓ Long-term PD plans
- ✓ Lifestyle goals
- ✓ Health improvement targets

Planning reduces uncertainty. Uncertainty increases stress.

**Final Thoughts**

Peritoneal Dialysis is not the end of life. It is a way to continue living.

With:

- ✓ Good planning
- ✓ Clean habits
- ✓ Emotional support
- ✓ Organized storage
- ✓ Hospital coordination

A patient can live safely and meaningfully for many years on PD.

Caregiving is not just about procedures. It is about preserving hope, dignity, and normalcy.

PD is treatment. Life is bigger than treatment.

And with proper discipline and compassion, both can move forward together.

# PART 8:
# PROFESSIONAL TOOLS

# Chapter 18: Standard Operating Procedure

**Step-by-Step Clinical Method for Safe Peritoneal Dialysis Exchange at Home**

This chapter provides a complete structured SOP (Standard Operating Procedure) for performing a Peritoneal Dialysis exchange safely at home.

This format is designed for:

- ✓ Caregivers
- ✓ Trained attendants
- ✓ Family members
- ✓ Home nurses

Follow this procedure exactly as trained by your PD unit. Never modify steps unless instructed by your doctor.

**SECTION 1: PRE-CHECK (Before Touching Any Equipment)**

Purpose: Ensure patient stability and equipment safety.

**1. Patient Pre-Check**

Confirm:

- ✓ No fever
- ✓ No abdominal pain
- ✓ No vomiting
- ✓ No breathlessness
- ✓ No severe swelling
- ✓ BP within acceptable range
- ✓ Weight recorded

If abnormal symptoms are present: → Contact doctor before proceeding.

**2. Environment Check**

Ensure:

- ✓ Clean designated PD area
- ✓ Good lighting
- ✓ No fan directly blowing
- ✓ Windows closed to prevent dust
- ✓ No pets in room
- ✓ No unnecessary people moving around

**3. Equipment Check**

Verify:

- ✓ Correct PD solution strength
- ✓ Correct volume
- ✓ Expiry date
- ✓ No leakage in bag
- ✓ Clear solution (no cloudiness)
- ✓ All clamps intact
- ✓ Minicap available
- ✓ Dressing materials ready (if needed)

Do not proceed if any item is damaged.

**SECTION 2: SETUP**

Purpose: Create sterile working environment.

**Step 1: Personal Preparation**

- ✓ Remove jewelry
- ✓ Wash hands using 6-step method
- ✓ Wear mask
- ✓ Wear sterile gloves

**Step 2: Table Preparation**

- ✓ Clean table with disinfectant
- ✓ Place clean newspaper or disposable sheet
- ✓ Arrange items in order of use
- ✓ Keep drain bag positioned lower than abdomen level
- ✓ Avoid touching sterile connection points.

**SECTION 3: DRAIN PHASE (Outflow)**

Purpose: Remove used dialysis fluid from abdomen.

**Step 1**

- ✓ Loosen bottom white minicap carefully.
- ✓ Avoid touching connection opening.

**Step 2**

- ✓ Connect green end from PD bag to catheter tubing.

**Step 3**

- ✓ Open white top cap as instructed.

**Step 4**

- ✓ Allow drain to start.
- ✓ Fluid should begin flowing downward into drain bag.

**Drain Monitoring**

Typical drain time: 10–20 minutes (varies per patient).

Fluid should flow steadily.

If slow, ask patient to change position.

Encourage mild movement or coughing if needed.

If no drain occurs: → Check for kinks. → Reposition patient. → If unresolved, contact doctor.

## SECTION 4: OBSERVE (Critical Safety Check)

Purpose: Inspect drained fluid before proceeding.

Hold drain bag over newspaper and check:

- ✓ Is fluid clear?
- ✓ Can you read print through it?

Normal fluid:

- ✓ Clear to pale yellow.

Abnormal findings:

- ✓ Cloudy → Possible infection
- ✓ Blood → Inform doctor
- ✓ White particles (fibrin) → Inform doctor (may need heparin)
- ✓ Foul smell → Report immediately

If abnormal: → Stop procedure. → Inform PD unit.

Do not ignore.

**SECTION 5: INFLOW PHASE (Filling)**

Purpose: Fill abdomen with fresh dialysis solution.

**Step 1**

Close drain clamp properly.

**Step 2**

Break green tube seals (as per training). Usually broken twice.

**Step 3**

- ✓ Open white clamp for inflow.
- ✓ Allow fluid to flow in.
- ✓ Some protocols mention 3-second white clamp timing for pressure regulation — follow your specific PD training instructions.

**During Inflow**

Monitor patient comfort.

Mild fullness is normal.

Severe pain is not normal.

If pain occurs: → Slow flow → Check positioning → Inform doctor if persistent

Inflow usually takes 5–10 minutes.

**SECTION 6: SEAL**

Purpose: Secure catheter after exchange.

**Step 1**

Close clamps securely.

**Step 2**

Disconnect tubing carefully.

**Step 3**

- ✓ Apply new sterile minicap.
- ✓ Ensure it is tightened properly.
- ✓ Never leave catheter open even briefly.

## SECTION 7: DISPOSE

Purpose: Safe waste management.

- ✓ Drain fluid into toilet (if advised).
- ✓ Dispose of used bag as per local medical waste guidance.
- ✓ Discard gloves and mask safely.
- ✓ Remove newspaper and discard.
- ✓ Clean table surface.
- ✓ Wash hands again after completion.

Hygiene does not end with exchange.

## SECTION 8: DOCUMENT FORMAT

Documentation is essential.

Maintain a daily PD record notebook.

**Sample PD Exchange Record Format**

Date:

Time of Exchange:

- ✓ PD Fluid Strength Used:
  Volume Used:
- ✓ Drain Volume:
  Drain Appearance: (Clear / Cloudy / Blood / Fibrin)
- ✓ Patient Symptoms:
  BP Before Exchange:
  Weight (if morning exchange):
- ✓ Any Issues During Drain:
  Any Issues During Inflow:

Signature/Name of Caregiver:

**Why Documentation Matters**

Documentation helps:

- ✓ Doctor adjust PD strength
- ✓ Detect early infection
- ✓ Monitor fluid balance
- ✓ Track trends over weeks

Memory fades. Written records protect patient safety.

**Complete Exchange Flow Summary**

- ✓ Pre-check patient and equipment
- ✓ Prepare clean setup
- ✓ Perform drain
- ✓ Observe fluid
- ✓ Perform inflow
- ✓ Seal securely
- ✓ Dispose safely
- ✓ Document completely

Follow this sequence every time. Never skip steps.

**Final Words**

This SOP is not just a checklist. It is a safety structure.

Each step protects:

- ✓ The peritoneal cavity
- ✓ The catheter
- ✓ The patient's health
- ✓ Your peace of mind

When done with discipline and calm attention, PD at home is safe and effective.

Professional care does not require a hospital building.

It requires trained hands, clean habits, and responsible documentation.

# Chapter 19:
# Printable Checklists & Logs

**Because Memory Can Fail — Paper Does Not**

In PD care, routine and discipline keep the patient safe. But even the most careful caregiver can forget small things when tired or stressed.

That is why written checklists are powerful.

They:

- ✓ Reduce mistakes
- ✓ Create consistency
- ✓ Help doctors review progress
- ✓ Build caregiver confidence
- ✓ Prevent emergencies

This chapter provides ready-to-use printable formats.

You can:

- ✓ Photocopy them
- ✓ Laminate them
- ✓ Keep them near the PD station
- ✓ Maintain them in a file

These are not just papers. They are safety tools.

## 1. PD EXCHANGE CHECKLIST

(To be used for every exchange)

You may print this as a one-page sheet and tick each box.

---

**PRE-CHECK**

☐ Patient feels well (no fever / no abdominal pain)

☐ BP checked (if required)

☐ Weight recorded (morning exchange)

☐ Clean exchange area ready

☐ No fan directly blowing

☐ Pets/children away

## EQUIPMENT CHECK

☐ Correct PD fluid strength
☐ Expiry date checked
☐ Bag clear (no cloudiness)
☐ No leakage or damage
☐ Minicap available
☐ Mask & gloves ready

## PERSONAL PREPARATION

☐ Hands washed (6-step method)
☐ Mask worn
☐ Sterile gloves worn

## DRAIN PHASE

☐ Minicap removed carefully
☐ Connection made without touching sterile points
☐ Drain started properly
☐ Drain completed fully

Drain Appearance:

☐ Clear
☐ Cloudy
☐ Blood
☐ Fibrin

If abnormal → Doctor informed? ☐ Yes ☐ No

## INFLOW PHASE

☐ Drain clamp closed
☐ Green tube broken correctly
☐ Inflow started smoothly
☐ Patient comfortable during inflow

**SEAL**

☐ Clamps closed properly

☐ New sterile minicap applied

☐ Catheter secured

---

**AFTER COMPLETION**

☐ Waste disposed safely

☐ Surface cleaned

☐ Hands washed again

☐ Exchange recorded in log

Signature: ___________Date & Time: _____________

---

## 2. EXIT SITE CARE CHECKLIST

(To be used daily)

---

**BEFORE STARTING**

☐ Hands washed

☐ Mask worn

☐ Sterile gloves worn

☐ Dressing items ready

---

**DURING CARE**

☐ Old dressing removed gently

☐ Exit site inspected

☐ No redness

☐ No swelling

☐ No discharge

☐ No pain

If abnormal → Doctor informed? ☐ Yes ☐ No

---

**CLEANING**

☐ Cleaned with prescribed solution (e.g., Benzodine)

☐ Cleaned from inside outward

☐ Area allowed to dry completely

---

**DRESSING**

☐ Ointment applied (if prescribed)

☐ Sterile gauze placed

☐ Transparent tape secured

☐ Catheter supported properly

Date: ____________Caregiver Name: ______________

---

## 3. DAILY MONITORING CHART

(To be maintained daily — one page per week recommended)

You may create a table like this:

| Date | Weight | BP | Fluid Intake (ml) | Urine Output (ml) | PD Volume | Drain | Swelling (Yes/No) | Appetite (Good/Average/Poor) | Remarks |
|---|---|---|---|---|---|---|---|---|---|

---

**Instructions for Use**

- ✓ Record weight every morning.
- ✓ Record BP at same time daily.
- ✓ Measure intake and output accurately.
- ✓ Write any unusual symptom in remarks.
- ✓ Bring this chart to every hospital visit.
- ✓ Doctors use this chart to adjust treatment safely.
- ✓ Incomplete records can delay proper decisions.

---

## 4. EMERGENCY REFERENCE SHEET

(Keep laminated near PD station)

This sheet should be simple and visible.

---

**CALL DOCTOR IMMEDIATELY IF:**

☐ Cloudy drain fluid
☐ Fever
☐ Severe abdominal pain
☐ Blood in drain fluid
☐ Severe breathlessness
☐ No drain output
☐ Sudden swelling
☐ Very high BP
☐ Very low BP with dizziness
☐ Continuous vomiting

---

**IMPORTANT CONTACT NUMBERS**

PD Doctor: ______________________________
PD Nurse: ______________________________
Hospital Emergency:
______________________________
Ambulance: ______________________________
Nearest Backup Hospital:
______________________________

**BASIC FIRST RESPONSE REMINDERS**

Stay calm.
Do not panic.
Do not self-medicate without advice.
Keep recent records ready.
Carry PD notebook to hospital.

**How to Organize These Logs at Home**

Keep:

- ✓ One file with plastic covers
- ✓ Separate section for each month
- ✓ Old records safely stored

Every month:

- ✓ Review patterns
- ✓ Check if weight is increasing
- ✓ Check if BP fluctuates
- ✓ Discuss trends with doctor
- ✓ Records show trends.

Trends show early warning signs.

**Why Printable Checklists Matter**

Many complications happen not because of lack of knowledge — but because of:

- ✓ Fatigue
- ✓ Distraction
- ✓ Overconfidence
- ✓ Routine becoming casual

Checklists bring discipline back. Even experienced nurses use checklists.

It is not weakness. It is professionalism.

**Final Words**

These printable tools turn your home into a structured care environment.

They:

- ✓ Reduce stress
- ✓ Increase confidence
- ✓ Improve communication with doctors
- ✓ Prevent avoidable complications

A well-maintained logbook is silent proof of responsible care-giving.

You are not "just helping." You are managing a clinical system at home.

And when done with discipline and care, it protects life every single day.

# Chapter 20: Frequently Asked Questions

**Simple Answers to Common Doubts**

When someone starts Peritoneal Dialysis (PD), questions do not stop.

Even after months of doing exchanges, new doubts arise. That is normal.

No question is silly when it concerns health.

This chapter answers some of the most common questions caregivers and patients ask.

---

## 1. How Long Does PD Continue?

Is This Temporary or Lifelong?

This is usually the first question families ask.

The honest answer is: It depends.

PD continues as long as:

- ✓ The peritoneal membrane works well
- ✓ Infections are controlled
- ✓ The patient tolerates it comfortably
- ✓ Doctor feels it is effective

For some patients, PD continues for many years.

For others, it may be used:

- ✓ Until kidney transplant
- ✓ Until medical condition changes
- ✓ Until membrane function reduces

PD is not automatically "lifelong."

It is a treatment option that works well for many people — sometimes for several years.

Regular hospital follow-ups help the doctor decide if PD is still effective.

Do not worry about "how many years."

Focus on:

- ✓ Good infection control
- ✓ Good nutrition
- ✓ Good monitoring

With discipline, PD can continue safely for a long time.

---

## 2. Can the Patient Bathe?

Yes — But Carefully

Bathing is allowed. But it must be done safely. The main concern is protecting the catheter exit site.

---

### General Bathing Guidelines

Avoid tub baths unless doctor permits. Prefer shower. Keep exit site protected.

Dry area thoroughly after bath.

Perform dressing after bathing if advised.

---

### Important Rules

- ✓ Do not soak in swimming pools without doctor approval.
- ✓ Avoid public hot tubs.
- ✓ Avoid bathing in unclean water.

After bathing:

- ✓ Gently pat dry.
- ✓ Do not rub the catheter site.
- ✓ Perform exit site dressing carefully.

If you notice redness after bathing, inform doctor.

Bathing improves hygiene — but careless bathing increases infection risk.

Balance is important.

---

## 3. When Should a Patient Switch to Hemodialysis (HD)?

This Decision Is Medical — Not Emotional

Sometimes families worry:
"Are we failing if we switch?" No.
Switching is not failure. It is a medical decision based on condition.

---

**Common Reasons for Switching to HD**

- ✓ Repeated severe peritonitis
- ✓ Peritoneal membrane not working effectively
- ✓ Frequent fluid overload despite adjustments
- ✓ Inadequate dialysis clearance
- ✓ Hernias that cannot be managed
- ✓ Patient preference

The doctor evaluates:

- ✓ Blood test results
- ✓ PD adequacy reports
- ✓ Infection history
- ✓ Overall health

Switching may be temporary or permanent.

---

**Emotional Side of Switching**

Patients may feel disappointed. They may think: "PD failed."
But that is not true.
PD may have served well for years.
Treatment plans change based on health needs.
Support the patient emotionally if such transition happens.
The goal is always: Safe and effective dialysis.

---

### 4. Can the Patient Travel Long-Term on PD?

Yes — with planning. Inform PD unit in advance.
Arrange supply delivery. Carry medical documents.
PD often allows more flexibility than hospital dialysis.

---

### 5. Can the Patient Exercise?

Yes, light exercise is usually encouraged. Walking is excellent.
Avoid heavy lifting (to prevent hernia).
Always confirm with doctor before starting new exercise.
Movement improves:

- ✓ Mood
- ✓ Appetite
- ✓ Circulation

---

**6. What If the Patient Feels "Normal"? Can Exchanges Be Reduced?**
No.
Even if the patient feels fine, exchanges must continue exactly as prescribed.
Feeling well means PD is working. Stopping or reducing without doctor advice can cause toxin buildup. Never adjust schedule on your own.

---

**7. Can PD Patients Eat Normally?**
Diet is controlled but not miserable.
With proper planning:

- ✓ Balanced meals
- ✓ Limited salt
- ✓ Controlled fluid
- ✓ Adequate protein

Food discipline protects long-term health.

---

**8. Is Occasional Abdominal Fullness Normal?**
Mild fullness during inflow is normal. Severe pain is not.
If pain persists or increases, contact doctor.

---

**9. How Do We Know PD Is Working?**
Signs PD is working:

- ✓ Stable blood reports
- ✓ Good appetite
- ✓ Controlled swelling
- ✓ Stable weight
- ✓ Clear drain fluid
- ✓ Controlled BP
- ✓ Regular lab tests confirm effectiveness.

---

**Final Thoughts**

Living with PD raises many questions. Do not hesitate to ask your PD nurse or doctor.

Clear communication prevents fear.

Remember:

No caregiver is expected to know everything. Learning happens gradually.

Confidence builds over time.

PD is not just a medical treatment. It is a partnership: Between patient, caregiver, and medical team.

With knowledge, discipline, and calm support, this partnership can remain strong for many years.

---

# About the Author
# 'GERARD ASSEY'

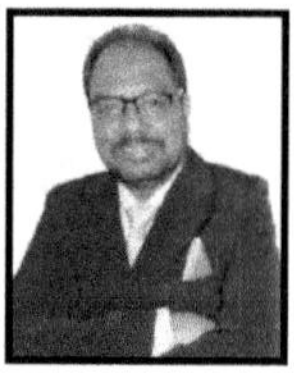

Gerard Assey is a Graduate in Economics, a PGD in Management (HRD) and holds a Doctorate in Leadership. Gerard holds several International Qualifications in Sales, Debt Collection, Training & Teaching, and is a 'Fellow' of the prestigious 'Institute of Sales & Marketing Management'-UK, a Certified NLP Practitioner, a 'Certified Trainer', an 'Accredited Management Teacher-Behavioral Sciences', a 'Certified Competency Facilitator', a 'Certified Management Consultant'- (the International credentials of a professional management consultant, awarded in accordance with global standards of the ICMCI); and a Certification from the University of Michigan in 'Successful Negotiation: Essential Strategies and Skills'

He is also a Member of the 'National Association of Sales Professionals' backed with several years experience in varied industries, both in India and Overseas. He also holds an 'Etiquette Consultant' Certification from the USA (by Sue Fox, Author of Best Seller: 'Business Etiquette for Dummies'. She has trained some of the top celebrities' world over). He was also a recipient of a scholarship for extensive training in Japan on 'Corporate Management for India'.

Gerard Assey is 'Founder & Chief Corporate Trainer' of the Group: '**Citius, Altius, Fortius Unlimited**'- an organization that **celebrated 20 years of Glorious Service** in 2021, focusing on 3 Core Competencies: **People. Performance. Profit**; in functional areas of Sales & Marketing, HR & Organizational Development, covering Recruitment, Training & Consultancy!

Having managed organizations with large Sales Forces in India & Overseas, his specialization cover extensive areas of Sales Training (All levels - Presentation, Negotiation, Key/ Strategic Accounts Management & Managerial Skills for all sectors), Bid Proposal/ Capture Planning/ Management Trainings, Retail Sales, Customer Service & Customer Retention Programs, Training for Prevention & Collection of Debt, Self & Personal Development Programs (Time Management, Teamwork & Team Building, Business Etiquette & Personal Grooming, Leadership & Managerial Skills, People Management Skills, Train-the-Trainer etc), including preparation of Custom-designed Business Manuals for Internal (HR, Induction, and Sales etc) & External use (Instruction, User Manuals).

Gerard has successfully conducted over 6495 Trainings & Workshops (as of Jan '26) all across India, Middle East, Africa, Europe & S.E. Asia. Besides public programs conducted regularly, both in India & Overseas, he has some of the top names as clients whom he services from Single Owners to large Public & Government undertakings, covering all sectors, for their in-house needs.

His website: www.CollectionSkills.com is the only one in this part of the world to be featured in the 'Collections & Credit Risk Magazine-USA' under 'Who's Who in Training' and ranks TOP, along with other websites listed below on most search engines.

**Gerard is author of 217 books already (Feb 2026),** all the books being available on all online platforms and outlets as E-books and Paperbacks

**A few of our business related books:**

1. Bite-sized Bits on Commonsense Management
2. Heart to Heart on Life's Principles'
3. How to become a Successful Manager
4. The Sales Professionals' Master Workbook of S.Y.S.T.E.M.S
5. The Professional Business Email Etiquette Handbook & Guide
6. The Professional Business Video-Conferencing Etiquette Handbook & Guide
7. Professional Presentation Skills
8. Exceptional Customer Service
9. Professional Tele-Marketing Skills
10. Professional Debt Collection Skills
11. The G.R.E.A.T. Sales & Service Workbook
12. Sales Training Advantage for Results (*The Ultimate Sales Training Manual to enable you stand out as a S.T.A.R.*)
13. CEO Daily Planner & Organizer
14. The Sales Professionals' Master Daily Planner
15. The Professional Debt Collector's Master Daily Planner
16. My Daily Planner & Organizer
17. MY EMERGENCY INFORMATION RECORD (Family Emergency & Peace of Mind Planner)
18. The Ultimate Therapist & Counselors Planner and Organizer
19. Building an Ethical Workplace
20. Managing Relationships at Work
21. Managing Business Meetings Effectively
22. Effective Delegation Skills
23. Goal Setting for Success
24. B2B Selling by Email
25. Professional Business Etiquette & Grooming
26. Dining Etiquette & Table Manners
27. Effective Networking Skills
28. Grooming, Etiquette & Manners for Teens, Young Adults & Future Leaders
29. Inter-Personal Skills
30. Get Ready, Get Hired!
31. Selling in a Recession

32. Effective Receivables Management in an Economic Downturn!
33. Real Estate & Property Sales Training
34. Credit Sales & Accounts Receivable Management
35. Selling Skills for Real Estate & Property Advisors
36. Take G.R.E.A.T. C.A.R.E!
37. Spa, Salon & Health Club Selling Skills
38. Selling Travel, Holiday & MICE Services
39. Selling Skills for Spa's, Salons & Health Clubs
40. Retailing in Salons & Spas
41. Selling Holiday, Vacation, Tours & Packages
42. The Power of Sales Referrals
43. Selling Luxury
44. Technical Selling Skills
45. Financial Advisors Sales Training
46. Dealing with Burnout at Work Monopolize Your Markets
47. Selling to Affluent Customers
48. Growing up with Grace
49. Financial Selling Skills
50. *The Effective Manager's Guide: Key Skills to Thrive*
51. From Aspiring to Inspiring: A Guide for New Managers on the Rise
52. The Power of Focus
53. Selling with Integrity: Sell Like Jesus The Perfect Role Model!
54. 31 Habits of Champions: Your 31-Day Journey to Greatness
55. Rejecting Grasshopper Talk: From Grasshopper to Giant-Killer-*Defeating Giants Daily!*
56. Navigate the AI-Powered Future of Bid & Proposals: Up-Skill to Stay Relevant with Alternative Career Paths & Opportunities
57. Hiring Sales Winners
58. Present with Impact
59. Success Unlocked: *Breaking Free from Habits that Hold You Back*
60. Complaints to Cheers, Feedback to Gold: Mastering Complaints Management
61. Thriving Together: *Cultivating Diversity, Equity, and Inclusion*
62. Coaching Skills for Sales Managers
63. Soaring to Success in Business & Leadership: Swifter, Higher, Stronger!

64. From Classroom to Podium: A Student's Guide to Powerful Public Speaking & Presentation Skills
65. Developing Self-Discipline
66. The CEO's 31-Day Power Plan: Unlocking Success through Essential Traits
67. Credibility Matters
68. A Winning Attitude
69. Bid & Proposal Management Using AI
70. Sales Forecasting: A Practical & Proven Guide to Strategic Sales Forecasting
71. Elevate & Energize: *50 Dynamic & Fun Activities for Peak Workplace Morale*
72. 'Sales SOS! Sales on Fire! *30 Days to Conquer Chaos & the Nightmares of Success!'*
73. Mastering Sales Managerial Skills: *Building High-Performing Teams & Driving Exceptional Results*
74. Eagle-Eyed Leadership: Unleashing the Power of 31 Lessons from Eagles
75. The Ultimate Employee Training Guide: *Training Today, Leading Tomorrow*
76. Being More Accountable at Work
77. Creating a Culture of Continuous Improvement
78. Effective Questioning & Listening Skills
79. The Power of Value Selling
80. The Growth Mindset
81. Mastering Professional Help Desk Skills
82. The Power to Lead with Empathy
83. Being Prepared: The Key to Unlocking Success
84. Youthful Spark-Youth Energizers, Activities and Games-Igniting the Fun in Youth
85. Ignite your Motivation for Success
86. Elevate Your Executive Presence: *Your Roadmap to Executive Excellence*
87. Smart Decisions: *Mastering Problem Solving with Strategic Solutions for Business Success*
88. Strategic Planning: *Developing and Implementing Strategic Plans to Achieve Long-Term Business Goals*
89. The Power of Stay Interviews
90. Developing G.R.I.T.
91. Adaptability
92. Diagnosis- *A Key Skill for Leadership*
93. The Burnout-Proof Salesperson: *The Master Guide to Preventing Stress & Burnout-* Strategies for Thriving in Sales

94. Learning from Failure: *Keys to Success*
95. Customer Success Management
96. Overcoming the Killers of Motivation
97. The C-Suite Code: *Mastering Skills for Executive Excellence'*
98. Dealing with Difficult Customers
99. Unlocking Your Potential: Mastering the Top 20 Life Skills for a Brighter Future
100. Nurturing Tomorrow's Leaders: *Essential Soft Skills Every Child Must Learn*
101. Lively & Fun Party Games for Seniors & Elders
102. Role Playing for Sales Champions: From Practice to Performance
103. Fun and Exciting Party Games for Kids
104. Case Studies for Sales
105. Role-Playing for Unbeatable Customer Service
106. Case Studies in Customer Service
107. Case Studies in Winning Negotiations
108. Case Studies in Management & Leadership
109. Case Studies in Human Resources & Talent Management
110. CEO Success Blueprint: The Essential Toolkit for CEOs and C-Level Executives
111. The Salesperson's Self-Coaching Guide: *Master Your Own Self-Coaching Plan for Success*
112. Overcoming Procrastination: *Your Ultimate Guide to Stop Delaying and Start Living Your Best Life*
113. When True Colors Are Exposed: *The Journey to Unmasking Humanity*
114. Life-Changing Habits for Teens: Teen Success Blueprint for a Bright Future
115. Workplace Stress-Free: *Proven Strategies to Thrive at Work and Beyond*
116. Objection Overruled: *The Ultimate Guide to Turning 'No' into 'Yes'"*
117. Building Strong Teams: *A Comprehensive Guide to Team Building*
118. Ethical & Moral Leadership in Business: *Eliminating Unethical Practices & Building a Culture of Trust & Integrity*
119. Rising Strong: Building Positive: High Self-Esteem for a Fulfilling Life-*A Practical Guide for Students, Employees, Leaders & Entrepreneurs*
120 The Cheerful Mindset: Cultivating a Joyful Outlook Everyday
121. Leading Through Crisis: Case Studies on Crisis

Management

122. Selling Beyond the Algorithms: *How to Harness AI, Automation & Human Intelligence to Win in Sales Today & Beyond*

***123.* PERITONEAL DIALYSIS CAREGIVER GUIDE**

Besides regularly contributing to business & trade journals, including international ones such as the 'Creative Training Techniques' and the 'Sales News' of the U.S.A, He is also a member of several prestigious bodies & trade associations, having participated in many Conferences & Workshops in India & Overseas.

Prior to his last assignment of leading & managing a large MNC as head, Gerard had a 3-year stint in the Middle East as a Consultant with a leading British Consultancy Firm.

As the past 'Official Country Representative' for the International Business Award- 'THE STEVIES'-(the business world's own Oscar) for about 4 years- he ensured a few Indian companies that qualify for the same every year!

Gerard can be contacted at:
Email: training@Sales-Training.in,training@CollectionSkills.com
Websites:

www.Sales-Training.in
www.EtiquetteWorks.in
www.CollectionSkills.com
www.RetailSalesTraining.in
www.SalesTrainingIndia.com
www.ManualPreparation.com
www.TrainingWithPuppets.com
www.FirstContactAcademy.com
www.SalesAndMarketingRecruiter.com

## Our TRAININGS that can help your team

- ✓ **Sales Effectiveness**: Selling Skills for any Sector: Service/ Logistics/ FMCG Realty/ Insurance & Finance/ Media/ SPA's, Health Clubs & Salons/ Key Account Management, Effective Negotiation Skills/ Bid & Proposal Management Skills/ Retail Sales Training: Any Sector (Auto, Jewelry, Clothing, Luxury etc)
- ✓ **Customer Service Skills**-Complaints Handling & Customer Retention
- ✓ **Debt Prevention & Collection Skills**
- ✓ **Etiquette & Grooming**
- ✓ **Leadership & Managerial Skills**
- ✓ **Self & Personal Development Skills**: Presentation Skills/ Effective Communication Skills/Business Proposal Writing Skills/ Problem Solving & Decision Making Skills/ Empowering Secretaries-The perfect PA! (For Secretaries & PA's)/ Effective Time Management/ Teamwork & Teambuilding/ P.R.I.D.E- **P**ersonal **R**esponsibility **I**n **D**elivering **E**xcellence

www.ingramcontent.com/pod-product-compliance
Ingram Content Group UK Ltd.
Pitfield, Milton Keynes, MK11 3LW, UK
UKHW021340190726
13845UKWH00027B/638

9 788199 878181